The
Good
Sleep
Guide

for
Neurodivergent Kids

Praise for *The Good Sleep Guide for Neurodivergent Kids*

"Dr. Melisa Moore has created the definitive guide every parent and clinician of neurodivergent kids has been waiting for. *The Good Sleep Guide for Neurodivergent Kids* brings together rigorous science, empathy, and lived experience in a way that feels both practical and profoundly human. As a sleep physician, I see families every day who are exhausted and searching for real-world solutions that actually work. This book delivers them with warmth, clarity, and compassion. Whether you're a parent, provider, or advocate, this is the resource that will finally help you understand your child's sleep and restore peace to the entire family."

— **Christopher J. Allen, MD**, "Sleep Dr. Chris," CEO and lead physician of Quality Sleep & Neurology PC

"This is the book I wish I could hand to every family who sits in my office exhausted and unsure of what to do next. Sleep is hard for so many neurodiverse kids, and parents are often left piecing together advice from a dozen places. This book finally brings it all together. It is practical, clear, and incredibly reassuring. Honestly, it feels like having a sleep psychologist in your pocket. I will be recommending it to the families I work with and encouraging them to order it, because it truly covers everything."

— **Willough Jenkins, MD**, child psychiatrist, associate professor, medical director, psychiatric emergency and consultation service, Rady Children's Hospital, University of California at San Diego

"As a pediatric sleep medicine specialist, I am delighted to endorse this wonderful book for parents. Dr. Moore, an experienced sleep psychologist, writes with both deep expertise and genuine heart, offering families guidance that is compassionate, practical, and grounded in real experience. Her ability to translate complex sleep science into clear, relatable advice makes this book an invaluable companion for any parent seeking to better understand and support their child's sleep."

— **Ignacio E. Tapia, MD, MS**, chief, division of pediatric pulmonology, Batchelor Professor of Cystic Fibrosis and Pediatric Pulmonology, University of Miami Miller School of Medicine

"Dr. Moore brings her mom experience to this gem of a book. It's easy to digest and chock-full of stories, Tuck-In Tips, and Pillow Points. I would recommend this quick read to all sleepy and stressed parents of neurodivergent kids."

— **Beth Ann Malow, MD, MS**, Burry Chair in Cognitive Childhood Development and professor of neurology and pediatrics at Vanderbilt University Medical Center

"Melisa Moore has written the book that so many parents and professionals have been waiting for — a definitive guide to improving sleep in neurodiverse children. Comprehensive, informed by research, and refreshingly accessible, it distills complex science into practical, easy-to-implement strategies. Most importantly, Dr. Moore's voice comes through with warmth and reassurance, making you feel as though she's right there beside you as you navigate your child's sleep challenges. This isn't just a helpful resource; it's a genuine lifeline (or at least a sleep-line) for exhausted, overwhelmed families searching for real solutions."

— **Christopher Willard, PsyD**, Harvard Medical School faculty member and author of more than twenty books, including *Feelings Are Like Farts* and *Growing Up Mindful*

"Dr. Melisa Moore is one of the world's foremost experts on sleep health in pediatric populations. Her command of the scientific literature provides the critical integrity, and her writing is accessible and practical. *The Good Sleep Guide for Neurodivergent Kids* should be on the bookshelf of every parent (and clinician) who is seeking solutions for the sleep problems families experience."

— **Michael A. Grandner, PhD**, director, Sleep and Health Research Program, associate professor of psychiatry, University of Arizona College of Medicine

"Melisa Moore has written a user-friendly, parent-reassuring, comprehensive, practical guide for parents of children with chronic sleep problems. Her calm, low-key style guides parents to help their children develop healthy, consistent sleep routines. Very importantly, she focuses on the special challenges of sleep for neurodiverse children. Every child psychiatrist and child specialist should keep a copy of this book in their office for ready reference and for recommendation to parents."

— **Kathleen Nadeau, PhD**, founder and director of The Chesapeake Center for ADHD, Learning and Behavioral Health; recipient of the 2025 CHADD Lifetime Achievement Award; and author of more than a dozen books related to ADHD, including *Still Distracted After All These Years: Help and Support for Older Adults with ADHD*

"At long last, here is the comprehensive sleep guide parents of neurodivergent children have been waiting for. With the perfect blend of science, professional expertise, and heart, Dr. Moore helps families understand both what's at the root of their child's sleep challenges and the steps they can take to help the whole family get the rest they need. We have referred countless parents and children to Dr. Moore over the years, and we have seen firsthand how effective her methods are."

— **Jennifer Waldburger, MSW**, and **Jill Spivack, LCSW**, coauthors of *The Sleepeasy Solution* and cofounders of Sleepy Planet Parenting

The Good Sleep Guide

for
Neurodivergent Kids

Science-Backed Strategies for Children and Teens with ADHD, Autism, and Other Neurodiversities

Melisa Moore, PhD

Foreword by Jodi A. Mindell, PhD

New World Library
Novato, California

New World Library
14 Pamaron Way
Novato, California 94949

The material in this book is intended for educational purposes only. No expressed or implied guarantee of the effects of the use of the recommendations can be given nor liability taken.

Text design by Tona Pearce Myers

Library of Congress Cataloging-in-Publication data is available.

First printing, March 2026
ISBN 978-1-955831-15-4
Ebook ISBN 978-1-955831-16-1
Printed in Canada

10   9   8   7   6   5   4   3   2   1

New World Library is committed to protecting our natural environment. This book is made of material from well-managed FSC®-certified forests, recycled materials, and other controlled sources.

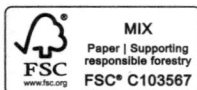

MIX
Paper | Supporting
responsible forestry
FSC
www.fsc.org   FSC® C103567

For my sons, who are each my favorite.

Neurodiverse and *neurodivergent* are often used synonymously, yet neither has a single, official definition. Various experts, advocacy groups, and individuals who consider themselves neurodiverse use the terms in their own ways. In this book, the terms are used interchangeably to refer to people with differences in executive functioning, communication, adaptability, and/or sensory processing. This is not meant to suggest that neurodivergent people are "less than." Rather, you're encouraged to define these differences in whatever way feels right to you. On the flip side, when you see the term *neurotypical* in this book, think of it as outside your definition of *neurodiverse*.

The families discussed in this book are fictional. They are composite portraits of people I've worked with and experiences I've had throughout my twenty years of practice. If you read an anecdote and think, "That must be my family!" know that it's not. Sleep problems are common among neurodiverse kids, and many families struggle with the same or similar issues.

Contents

Part 1: Neurodiverse Sleep

Part 2: Improving Sleep in Neurodiverse Kids

Foreword

If you are the parent of a neurodivergent child with (or even without) sleep issues, congratulations on finding this book! You have come to the right place. *The Good Sleep Guide for Neurodivergent Kids* provides well-researched, practical information to help everyone in your family get a good night's sleep.

The term *neurodivergent* casts a wide net and includes children and adolescents with differences that include autism spectrum disorder (ASD), attention-deficit/hyperactivity disorder (ADHD), genetic syndromes, and learning differences. Unfortunately, sleep problems are so common among neurodivergent children that they have almost become expected, and in many cases even accepted. Children with neurodiversities often have a difficult time falling asleep, may wake up for long stretches during the night, or can even seem to need less sleep than other children their age. Sadly, sleep issues, in turn, have negative effects on neurodiversities. For example, children who do not get the sleep they need may have a more difficult time focusing and/or regulating their emotions. *The Good Sleep Guide for Neurodivergent Kids* covers all of these topics, including the basics behind sleep, why sleep is important, what factors affect sleep, and ways to manage and improve your child's sleep and your own sleep. Also, this information and advice is universal and can help you manage sleep challenges faced by neurotypical children.

Dr. Melisa Moore is a world-renowned expert in improving

sleep in children, especially those who are neurodivergent. She has advised countless parents, trained scores of healthcare providers, and contributed to the growing body of science on childhood sleep. She has spent her entire career considering how neurodevelopmental differences — especially autism — affect sleep patterns and how to tailor interventions to help each child and each family.

What's more, Dr. Moore has not only devoted her professional life to improving children's sleep, but she has lived this issue! Her son, diagnosed with autism as a young child, has been one of her greatest teachers. Like her clients, she has navigated bedtime struggles, middle-of-the-night wakings, and sensory sensitivities. She has lived the exhaustion, the uncertainty, and the trial-and-error process that so many parents know all too well. I have had many conversations with her about her son's struggles with sleep and how to manage his unique needs. These experiences have led her to develop a deep level of understanding and compassion, which elevates her scientific understanding of these topics with personal experience only a parent can have.

I have been fortunate to know Dr. Moore both personally and professionally. We worked together for almost two decades at the Sleep Center at Children's Hospital of Philadelphia. She is one of the best sleep doctors I know, and she is one of only a few pediatric specialists to receive a Diplomate in Behavioral Sleep Medicine. This is an impressive credential bestowed by the Board of Behavioral Sleep Medicine to behavioral health providers who meet specific educational and clinical experience requirements and pass a specialty examination. She truly understands the needs of children and their families. Dr. Moore writes as an expert *and* a mother.

The Good Sleep Guide for Neurodivergent Kids provides parents and other caregivers with the tools they need to help everyone in the family get a good night's sleep or, at the very least, a better night's sleep! And this book recognizes the fact that different families need different strategies. You won't find rigid, one-size-fits-all recommendations. Instead, Dr. Moore offers a framework to help you figure out what works best for your child and your family's circumstances. She gives you the tools to understand sleep, observe patterns that affect your child, and respond to what works best for your child's needs. And she does this both as an expert in children's sleep and as someone who has walked the walk. She understands that the most effective solutions may not be the "standard" recommendations but those that work for your child and your family — whether that includes screen time before bed to settle in, leaving a snack by the bedside for middle-of-the-night hunger, or integrating your child's particular sensory needs into their bedtime routine. *The Good Sleep Guide for Neurodivergent Kids* provides both an understanding of the science of sleep and the lived wisdom of an experienced mom. You are not alone in this journey.

Dr. Moore's goal has always been to educate the world about sleep and provide the gift of a good night's sleep to every family and child, especially neurodivergent children. Whether you're reading this book at 9 p.m. after bedtime or at 2 a.m. in the quiet (or not-so-quiet) dark, you will find the practical guidance, tools, and genuine understanding you need. This combination of expertise and lived experience is the reason Dr. Moore has helped thousands of families, and it is why this book can give you and your family the gift of a good night's sleep.

Jodi A. Mindell, PhD
Associate Director, Sleep Center,
Children's Hospital of Philadelphia
Professor, Saint Joseph's University
Author of *Sleeping Through the Night: How Infants, Toddlers, and Their Parents Can Get a Good Night's Sleep*
and *A Clinical Guide to Pediatric Sleep*

Preface

I'm tired.

I'm tired as I write this because I've been woken up for the last very many nights around 2 a.m. by my son Henry, who has critically important questions that cannot wait even one second: What color is the rain on Mars? Do snakes have butts? Is heaven above the clouds or below the clouds? What if Abraham Lincoln was born with his clothes on?

Huh?

The answer to all of these is: I have no idea and please, *please* go back to sleep.

My oldest son, who was eleven when I wrote this book, has autism spectrum disorder (ASD), attention-deficit/hyperactivity disorder (ADHD), and the kind of seemingly random sleep problems that tend to exist side by side with neurodiversity.

I am a psychologist specializing in children's sleep, and I was nearly ten years into this career before I had my first child. At that point, I had already done a lot of book learning, training, thinking, studying, writing, researching, and talking about sleep. I had already seen thousands of children and had experience with all different kinds of families. I thought I knew a lot about sleep. Then, boom! I became the parent of a child born with ASD, and I pretty much instantly grasped how truly precious sleep is and how challenging it can be to make it better. Prior to this, I knew that the recommendations I gave families might be hard to try at home.

Then I learned firsthand that "hard" doesn't begin to scratch the surface. At home I received a brand-new education in the challenges of parenting a neurodiverse kid, one whose sleep problems aren't anyone's fault or caused by bad habits. They occur with neurodiversity.

That is the reason I'm writing this book. If someone like me — someone with a PhD in pediatric behavioral sleep medicine, professional colleagues I can turn to, and access to a wealth of resources — can still find managing the sleep of my neurodivergent child unbelievably confusing and difficult, then I know it must be exponentially tougher for every other parent on the planet. I use the term *parent* in the broadest sense — to refer to any and all caregivers, whatever their actual relationship or title. When I say *parent*, I also mean grandparents, aunts, uncles, second cousins once removed, foster parents, stepparents, teachers, neighbors, therapists, and anyone else who cares for a neurodiverse child or teen with sleep problems.

Similarly, by *bed* and *bedroom*, I mean the surface and room where your child sleeps. By necessity or choice, some families all sleep in different rooms, and some families all share one bed. Some siblings share a room. Some kids sleep at different houses on different nights. Your child does not have to have their own bed or bedroom for their sleep to improve.

I hope this book helps your family to get better sleep and that it validates your struggles and experience. I might be a "sleep expert," but I am right there with you.

I want you to feel seen and understood, but I also recognize that my personal experience is different than yours. I've been in plenty of conversations with well-meaning people who compare their neurotypical child's struggles with mine, and at times I have to suppress some eye rolls. And I've worked with enough families to know that, while my family may be floating around the same sea of neurodiversity as theirs, each family with a neurodiverse child is in their own particular boat. People talk about neurodiversity and particularly ASD as a spectrum, and it's difficult to give sleep advice to everyone on that spectrum. There are families whose toddler has boundless energy at bedtime but sleeps through the night, whose preschooler is happily awake and singing for three hours in the middle of each night, and whose ten-year-old child has never slept through the night. My son requires moderate support, and his sleep issues include long wakings, restlessness, constant questions, middle-of-the-night hunger, and dependence on a specific koala eye mask. Other children may be visually impaired, have ADHD with racing thoughts and ideas, engage in unsafe nighttime behaviors, start every single day at 4 a.m., need special stretchy sheets, or be unable to explain why they can't sleep or what they need, leaving parents unsure how to help.

Throughout this book, I try to acknowledge that my own personal experience won't match yours. I don't and can't know your particular struggles. But I've worked with families with neurodiverse children across the entire spectrum, and one thing I've learned is that most sleep problems are similar across the breadth of that spectrum. The underlying processes and the reasons things go haywire are generally the same for most neurodiverse people. I may not know what life is like in your boat, but I think I can help.

I also know something else: The free time of a parent with a neurodiverse child is minimal. I've tried to write this book so that it can be read quickly and easily. Then, at the end of each chapter, I provide "Tuck-In Tips" that summarize the important points. This is followed by a "Pillow Point," which is what I consider the chapter's single most important takeaway. If exhaustion is getting the better of you, skip to the end of each chapter.

In this book, I describe ideal sleep habits and discuss where the ideal meets the real. Definitions of healthy sleep are flexible, and I bring this to life through stories as well as science. I offer adaptations, adjustments, and ideas that I've learned from research, friends, colleagues, my family, and the families I've been lucky enough to work with. I focus primarily on treatments with the most scientifically proven effectiveness, but at times I step outside the box to describe ideas without the same research foundation. The advice in this book won't apply to everyone, and you don't have to read it all, either. Read what applies to you, skip around, and come back to it later if you're too sleepy to keep reading. Do what works for you.

I'm hopeful that — armed with new information, strategies for improving sleep, ideas for coping with a difficult sleeper, and real-life examples — you and your child will soon be on your way to a better night's sleep and brighter days ahead.

PART 1

Neurodiverse Sleep

Chapter 1

In the Beginning

The sleep deprivation that comes with being a first-time parent is shocking. When it is prolonged past the newborn stage, it can be devastating. I've told the following unflattering story about myself many times because I think it speaks to the harshness and confusion of new parenthood. I went through a multiday labor that ended with a C-section. After surgery, the nurse came in to tell me I needed to breastfeed or pump every two hours. I sheepishly said that after everything I'd been through, I really needed a longer stretch of sleep to recover. I cried as I explained how worried I was about dropping my baby because my reaction time would be terrible after days of sleep deprivation. I told her that I knew this because of my job.

She looked at me, rolled her eyes, and walked out of the room, saying, "Welcome to motherhood." Though my concerns were genuine, I was obviously clueless.

On paper and as a professional, I was well aware of the impact of poor sleep. I've worked with adults who have inconsistent, insufficient sleep because of their jobs: medical residents, heart-transplant surgeons, military special forces personnel, rock stars, actors, you name it. Yet I was stunned at how awful the actual experience of sleep deprivation feels day after day. The lack of sleep parents (especially mothers) in the newborn phase endure is astonishing. This is especially true during the first three to four months of a child's life regardless of neurodiversity. Why?

To break it down, babies' bodies aren't primed to sleep at night for consolidated periods until about three to four months of age.[1] Hormones such as melatonin and cortisol aren't synchronized with changes in body temperature and blood pressure. At birth, these processes are independent instruments and not yet playing together. There isn't much we can do to hurry the orchestra along. It's a good idea to differentiate night and day with light, sound, activity, and food, but that's really all we can do. At night, keep the environment dark, quiet, and calm, and during the day, expose your baby to natural sunlight as well as typical daytime noises and activities.

During those first months, get all the help you can so that *you* get more sleep. What is possible or works best will depend on your specific situation. Maybe ask a friend to come over for an hour a few times a week so you can nap, have your parents or in-laws come for an extended visit, or split the night into two shifts between partners. Keep any feeding or pumping supplies next to the bed to minimize middle-of-the-night interruptions. Commiserate with and get ideas from other parents.

Early Sleep Patterns and Neurodiversity

Sleep problems are even more common when a child has a medical problem or neurodevelopmental condition. In fact, disrupted sleep or unusual sleep patterns may be an early indicator that something is different.[2] There isn't one definitive reason why sleep problems are more prevalent in neurodivergent children and teens, though I describe many possibilities in chapter 4. My husband still frequently asks, "Why did Henry wake up last night?" There is no magic answer, and I remind him that it is what it is; we just have to get through it.

In my experience, after the impact of the newborn experience wears off, if a parent thinks something is unusual, it's best to take that feeling seriously. Since the sleep challenges of typical infants can themselves be hellish, it can be hard to evaluate the advice you get from well-meaning friends and family members. Even good suggestions from sleep coaches and pediatricians often don't address sleep issues that go above and beyond typical parent struggles. When I first started working in sleep, I was shouting from the rooftops about the importance of good sleep for development and mental health. As years have passed and Covid added uncertainty and chaos, I've noticed families sometimes defer developmental evaluations; they want to wait until their child's sleep is fixed because they *do* recognize the importance of sleep. Trust your caregiving gut. If you suspect that your child might have a neurodevelopmental or medical condition impacting sleep, don't wait. While it's true that sleep impacts the symptoms of ADHD, ASD, and other neurodiversities, it is perhaps even more true that neurodiversity affects sleep.

Should you start with a sleep physician, a psychologist, or a psychiatrist? Early intervention, a behavior therapist, or a speech pathologist? The correct answer is to start somewhere, anywhere, because there is no correct order. Many families don't have access to specialists. They receive care through a general pediatrician, primary-care physician, family-medicine physician, or nurse practitioner, which is a good place to start. Ask for recommendations from physicians, teachers, friends, and/or family members. Typically, states run evaluation programs for all ages. If your child is younger than three, connect with your state's early-intervention program.[3] If your child is older than three, call any elementary school in your district, even if your child doesn't go to that school. Someone will likely know who to call for services in your child's age range. I recommend getting started with any kind of educational, medical, developmental, or psychological evaluation sooner rather than later for two reasons.

First, as I mentioned, sleep problems can be one of the first signs of neurodiversity.[4] In fact, sleep problems were part of the diagnostic criteria for ADHD until 1987.[5] Today, sleep problems are no longer considered a core feature of any neurodevelopmental condition; they are considered a separate, coexisting condition — a comorbidity riding sidecar. That said, sleep problems are incredibly common in people with neurodiverse conditions. The other reason not to wait is because, in the United States, there aren't enough child development specialists, developmental pediatricians, child/adolescent mental health providers, pediatric sleep physicians, or pediatric sleep psychologists. Many of these in-demand providers have long waitlists, and my suggestion is to get on more than one. You can always cancel if the time comes and you no longer need an appointment.

Differentiating typical sleep problems from those associated with neurodivergence often requires the help of a specialist, even if you are a specialist. This was true for me. I look back and I can't believe I didn't recognize that my child was neurodiverse sooner. I knew he was special, and I loved his quirkiness — I still do. One of his sleep idiosyncrasies as a baby was repeating new words over and over until he drifted off. When he was about nine months old, he would repeat "tickle, tickle, tickle" without stopping for twenty to thirty minutes until he fell asleep. It was very sweet. Now he makes noises or sings songs that are less sweet ("All Star" by Smash Mouth is a current favorite), and they are too loud for me to sleep through.

I suspected something was different about Henry's development at about age two, and though I pulled every possible string I had, it was several months before I could get him an evaluation with a developmental pediatrician. I also scheduled an evaluation with our state's early-intervention program and with a play therapist. The only way I can describe this time is that I was in an emotional black hole and blindly reaching in every direction for help. For me, knowing something was different but not knowing what it was or what to do was the worst feeling I have ever experienced.

Every waking second, my brain was consumed by worry and nausea. It took about nine months of hard-core seeking to find experts who could give me advice that would help Henry. This was not because people didn't want to be helpful. It just took time to move up on the waitlists, get an evaluation, be told we needed a different specialist or evaluation, and find the right experts. I am forever grateful to Henry's long-term speech therapist, Susan, who was the first person to say, "I work with kids like Henry, and this is the right place. I can help him." Hearing that lifted me up. Gradually, I found a behavior therapist, an occupational therapist, a developmental pediatrician, and a diverse and accepting preschool. This group of providers was my first "team Henry."

On the playground outside of Susan's speech-therapy practice, I found other moms who are still my lifeline. This group of moms gets a part of me that no one else can understand. They helped me get through the initial paradigm shift: from expecting to be the parent of a neurotypical child to becoming the parent Henry needed. Through these moms I found my city's special-needs Facebook group, and despite being a Luddite at social media, I've reached out this way wherever I've lived. This is the most helpful advice I can give, whenever your journey begins: Find your people and create your team.

Keep in mind that finding the right team members takes time. Providers assigned to you by early-intervention, school, and state programs can almost always be switched if they aren't a good match. The first therapist assigned to us from state early intervention walked in the door squealing, "OMG, I love special needs!" She was just out of college and trying to be enthusiastic, but after a few months, Henry wasn't making progress working with her. They just didn't click. Then one day a friend asked me why I hadn't requested a new therapist. The reason was only that I had no idea that was possible. After requesting a switch, we had a series of amazing behavior therapists that Henry did click with, and I could see him growing and learning after the first few sessions.

Not only has Henry learned new skills from his therapists, I have, too. I'm a different psychologist, both from personal experience and from watching Henry's incredibly skilled providers. When Henry was first diagnosed with ASD, I didn't share what was going on with many of my colleagues or with the families I worked with at the clinic. Initially, I felt that it was unprofessional to tell patients and families that I was also experiencing what they were going through. I didn't want my clinical work helping others to become focused on me. Yet even then, I understood from personal experience how valuable it feels to be seen by someone who knows.

The first time I talked about my own family's challenges with neurodiversity and sleep in a professional context was a few years ago, after I moved to California. I was speaking at a conference on autism and comorbid conditions aimed at both families and providers. The presentation before mine, about independent housing for neurodiverse kids, was given by a mom who was in the throes of it. Hearing her speak about her own experience was incredibly powerful and gave me such hope for Henry's future. During my talk on sleep, I decided to do the same thing. I unexpectedly veered off script to say that I was the mom of a neurodiverse kid who was also living these sleep problems. After that talk, I transitioned (inside and out) from a sleep specialist with a niche in neurodiversity to a sleep specialist with lived experience in the sleep problems that often accompany neurodiversity.

Today, if I think it's therapeutic, within my professional boundaries, and respectful of my neurodivergent son and his brother, I share my family's experiences. This shift is also part of what inspired me to write this book. And the feedback I've received from families has been overwhelmingly positive. I want families of neurodivergent kids to know that we are in this together.

Tuck-In Tips

- For the first months of your child's life, get as much help as you can so you can sleep.
- The elements needed for our bodies to establish a consistent circadian rhythm are not coordinated until about four months of age.
- To help your newborn's emerging circadian rhythm, differentiate night and day with light, sound, and activity levels.
- At any time, if you have concerns about your child's development, seek evaluations and get on waitlists. Don't wait, hoping your child will grow out of their sleep problem first.
- Find your people and build your child's team — of professionals, friends, family, and people who share your experience.

Pillow Point

In person and through online communities, seek support and advice from people who are going through what you are going through, whether it is coping with the sleep deprivation that comes with a newborn or your child undergoing a developmental evaluation.

Chapter 2

What Causes Sleep?

My son Henry was a great napper until almost age three. I even scheduled my work around these naps during those years. If he didn't have a nap, Henry would fall asleep during his occupational therapy at home, and meltdowns were common. In the months after Henry turned three, he started taking longer to fall asleep in the afternoons, and his schedule shifted later. Eventually, he woke up from his nap around 5 p.m., and as a result, his 7:30 p.m. bedtime became a disaster. After a long nightly struggle, Henry would finally fall asleep around 10 p.m. I kissed my daytime work schedule goodbye until I was able to find help, and I started shortening Henry's naps. This beautiful nap situation fell apart because of sleep pressure, one of the main drivers of sleep.

During the summer of this shift, we were on vacation with my in-laws, staying in a beautiful old house without air-conditioning. Our bedroom was filled with sun due to the lovely light-filtering shades on the windows. For nighttime and for naps, falling asleep in this brightness was challenging for my toddler at best and non-existent at worst. I got so desperate that I scrounged around until I found an industrial-sized role of aluminum foil and made blackout shades for the bedroom windows. It worked like a charm, and even though it felt like summertime in the desert, Henry slept peacefully in the dark and under the fan. Those DIY blackout curtains saved the day because they prevented the sun from cueing Henry that it was *not* time to sleep. They kept his circadian rhythm, another critical aspect of sleep, aligned with day and night.

Throughout Henry's early years, for naps and at night, sleep was impossible for our entire family without Blue, Henry's hungry-caterpillar-patterned, minky-textured, taggy blanket I had bought on Etsy. Literally, there will never be another Blue. When I recognized how pivotal Blue was to Henry's sleep, I tried to find another. Neither the original seller nor any of the 6,423 other sellers of taggy blankets on Etsy could make an identical one. Even if they could, how would we have replicated Blue's distinct dried-baby-saliva, laundry-soap, strawberry-yogurt-puff smell? Keeping track of Blue's whereabouts took a significant chunk of my brain because I was obsessed with sleep, and AirTags didn't exist then.

Once, when my best friend was visiting for the weekend from New Jersey, Henry hid Blue in her boot. When she left, Blue accidentally went with her for an impromptu vacation to South Orange. I panicked and immediately searched again for a new Blue on Etsy. When that failed, I tearfully called my friend, begging her to FedEx the blanket immediately. My more-experienced-at-parenting friend thought my urgency was extreme. I didn't care. Because it was, of course, a holiday weekend, "overnight express" took two very rough, tear-stained, sleepless nights. I took a video of the moment when Henry opened the FedEx box and realized Blue was inside. He radiated pure joy, and I still occasionally watch that video if I need a lift.

Henry had a sleep association with Blue, and he needed that blanket in order to fall asleep. He eventually transferred that association to a striped cat named Paul, and later to a blue plushy letter I named Cyan. Today, a dinosaur neck pillow and a silky koala eye mask have also joined the crew.

Sleep pressure, circadian rhythms, and sleep associations are the things that cause us to feel sleepy, fall asleep, and stay asleep regardless of how old we are and no matter where we are on the spectrum of neurodiversity. While these three processes may operate in uncommon ways for kids who are developing differently, the same underlying mechanisms are at work.

Sleep Pressure

Sleep pressure is what it sounds like. Our need for sleep builds just like steam in a pressure cooker. Our bodies are always trying to get to a balanced state, so the further away we are from the last time we slept, the more we need sleep. When we wake in the morning, theoretically we shouldn't need more sleep (unless we were woken at 4 a.m. by a child scream-singing "We Are the Champions"). As the day goes on, sleep pressure steadily builds until it reaches a threshold — an invisible line that signals to our brain that it's time for the pressure to be released. Sleep is the only way to release that pressure.

Stimulant medications and caffeine may temporarily prevent dozing off during a boring Zoom meeting, but they do not take away the underlying drive for sleep. However, taking a quick nap or sleeping late on the weekend *does* take away sleep pressure, just like nighttime sleep does. So, for children who have trouble falling asleep or staying asleep at night, extra daytime sleep may not be good. Younger kids need naps because their sleep pressure builds more quickly, but after kindergarten age or so, naps will take away the sleep pressure that is needed for a full night's sleep. Unless your child is of napping age or has a medical reason to sleep during the day, they should be awake all day long. This may mean talking to teachers and daycare providers about shortening or eliminating that daytime nap and/or waking your child if they fall asleep in class.

Our Circadian Rhythm

The circadian rhythm is our body's internal sleep/wake clock. Exposure to morning sunlight is the most effective way to nudge the circadian clock to stay awake during the day and fall asleep at night. Neurodiverse kids can be especially sensitive to changes in light (no thanks, daylight saving time!), and getting direct, natural sunshine in the morning is a key part of keeping that circadian clock running smoothly. At the opposite end, if a child is a 4 a.m. early riser, restrict light and keep those blackout shades down until it is a reasonable time to be morning. For me, that's 6 a.m.

The circadian rhythm is intertwined with everyone's favorite sleep hormone, melatonin. Melatonin is turned *off* by sunlight and by the specific kind of light emitted from electronics. Does this mean everyone has to turn off electronics two hours before bedtime? Not necessarily. For some kids, using electronics at night can trick the brain into thinking it's day, making it more difficult to fall asleep. For others, using electronics is less of an issue when it comes to sleep. Also, it's not a problem to leave on a nightlight or a reading light at night. This doesn't have the same impact as sunlight or electronics.

Circadian cells exist all over the body. Aside from the visual system, the greatest concentration of circadian cells is in the gastrointestinal system. Thus, sleep can be improved by scheduling a child's mealtimes during the day at consistent, typical intervals: breakfast in the morning, lunch midday, and dinner in the evening.

With neurodiverse kids, this can be tricky if (1) your child is fed by feeding tube, (2) they get hungry at night because they haven't eaten enough during the day (for example, because of an appetite-suppressing medication), and/or (3) your family's schedule makes regular mealtimes impossible. If your child is tube fed, talk to your child's doctor about avoiding overnight feeds or at least decreasing them if possible. In addition to giving the circadian cells the wrong information, tube feeds can cause some tummy troubles that interfere with sleep. If your child doesn't eat enough during the day for whatever reason, nighttime hunger can be a dilemma. I'm not talking about requests for popcorn or extra ice cream when it's time to brush teeth and turn the lights off. Those are delay tactics, curtain calls, silly talk. Genuine hunger at night does interfere with sleep, so a bedtime snack might be an important part of your child's sleep routine.

No matter what the sleep issue is, balance the ideal with your family's real by starting with this question: What allows everyone in the house (including you) to get as much sleep as possible? That might involve bending parenting standards a bit.

For instance, starting around kindergarten, Henry had night-time hunger pangs that disturbed his (and my) sleep. Initially, I tried to provide healthy protein snacks, but they were left uneaten. Instead, Henry woke with an urgent need for strawberries, Jell-O, or dried kiwi. He sometimes cried with hunger as I raced to cut grapes in half. What helped us all sleep through the night more often has been this routine: At bedtime I put an orange Jell-O, a spoon, a banana with scissors (because he likes to open the banana that way), a plastic bag of Oreos, and one or two bowls of fruit on the dresser beside his bed. Is this ideal for his teeth? No way. Absolutely not, and I apologize to the dentists and dental hygienists out there, especially those who work at my kids' dental practice. Is this ideal for sleep? No, but remember: We are aiming for the place where the ideal meets the real. This is that place for my family. It's not a perfect system. I am still sometimes woken up to be told that the banana is too big or too mushy or that the spoon needs to go in the sink. But I don't have to go down to the kitchen at 2 a.m. only to find that we don't have any bananas or we have every color of Jell-O but orange.

Sleep Associations and Sleep Cycles

We all have sleep cycles that include non-rapid eye movement (NREM) and rapid eye movement (REM) sleep. Each sleep cycle has four stages, and this gets repeated several times during the night, as shown in the illustration that follows.

Typical Sleep Cycle

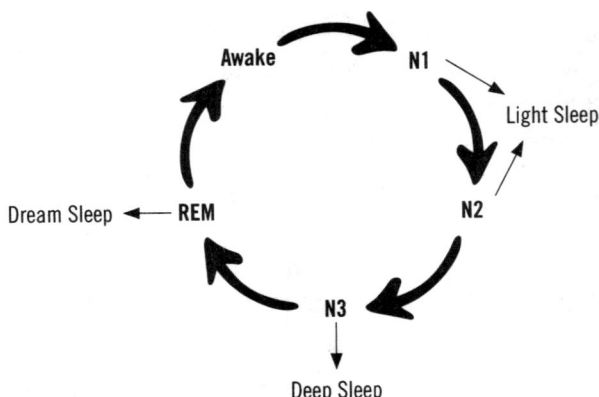

When we first fall asleep, we go from awake to very light sleep, the N1 stage, which lasts about one to seven minutes. Our brains and bodies slow down, but we are still easy to wake.

The next stage, N2, is also considered light sleep. Body temperature drops, muscles relax, eyes stop moving, and heart rate, breathing, and brain activity slow down. N2 lasts about ten to twenty-five minutes during the first sleep cycle, and it gets longer as the night goes on. As the sleep cycle progresses, it becomes harder to wake someone up, and by N3, deep sleep (also called slow wave or delta sleep), it is generally pretty difficult. This is the stage where we can get toddlers out of the car, change their pj's, and put them into bed without them waking. Each period of N3 sleep lasts about twenty to forty minutes during the early part of the night. This is when the body gets restorative sleep, when it recovers and grows. I tell children and teens that if they want to be taller, they should get good sleep because that is when their growth hormone is secreted! N3 sleep also boosts the immune system and helps other important body functions. Even if we are sleep-deprived or we don't get enough sleep one night, the brain will prioritize getting N3 sleep first. We get the deepest sleep in the first half of the night, and during the second half of the night, N3 gets shorter as REM sleep gets longer.

We first go into REM sleep about sixty to ninety minutes after we fall asleep. During REM, our brain activity increases almost to the same level as when we are awake. At the same time, our muscles are paralyzed so that we can't act out our dreams. The exceptions to that are breathing muscles and eye muscles (which move rapidly, thus the name). At the beginning of the night, REM may only be a few minutes long, while at the end of the night, it can last about an hour. Though deep sleep (N3) is considered the most restorative stage, REM sleep is important for brain functions such as learning, memory, and creativity.

After the REM stage, we briefly wake up before starting a new sleep cycle. Most of the time, we are so efficient at getting ourselves back to sleep that we don't even know we ever woke. For everyone, child or adult, nighttime wakings are a normal part of the sleep cycle.

When I hear that a child is waking up frequently during the night, I know that the most likely cause is actually that they can't get *back* to sleep after the brief waking at the end of a sleep cycle. This doesn't necessarily happen with every single waking. It's unpredictable — sometimes children do return to sleep independently, or on their own. But when they can't, children cry, yell, or somehow wake their parents. This is likely because of a sleep association. Sleep associations are the things our brain connects with sleep (like Blue for Henry), and those associations are present *all night long*. Whatever is needed to go from awake to asleep at bedtime is what is needed to get back to sleep easily during a normal night waking.

This is a lightbulb moment for most people, and I tell every parent whose child struggles to sleep the same thing: *If your child doesn't have what they need to calm down and fall asleep at bedtime, it will be harder for them to get back to sleep during those normal night wakings.* So, if your child falls asleep listening to Coldplay lullabies, reading a book, watching TV, drinking a bottle, looking at a toy aquarium, or being rocked, they may wake you up because they need that same activity or object in order to easily get back to sleep again. Without it, the sleep cycle is interrupted.

As a psychologist, some of my favorite sleep problems are sleep associations, since they are almost always changeable. First of all, we develop sleep associations when we are wide awake, not when we are two seconds away from sleep. If we rock our child until they are drowsy and then put them in the crib, then rocking becomes their sleep association, and they will have a harder time returning to sleep during the night without rocking. So create a sleep association that your child can keep with them the whole time they are sleeping. I've helped children with every sleep association you can imagine — touching running water, twirling mom's hair, touching dad's earlobe, patting grandpa's beard, listening to Toby Keith, kicking the wall, hugging a stuffed ostrich, spinning toy car wheels...whatever. Ideally, electronics should not be sleep associations, but if the iPad is the only way your neurodiverse child will stay in bed long enough to calm down, it won't ruin their life. Once your child does develop a helpful sleep association to an object, buy several of that thing and rotate them (for more, see chapter 13).

Don't be like me and create a sleep association to a one-of-a-kind Blue.

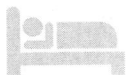

Tuck-In Tips

- Three processes control sleep for everyone: sleep pressure, circadian rhythm, and sleep associations.
- **Sleep pressure:** This is the need for sleep, which builds throughout the day and is reduced only by sleep.
  - **Tip:** Avoid all daytime sleep, unless your child is at an appropriate age for napping.

- **Circadian rhythm:** This is our body's internal clock.
  - **Tip:** Get sunlight in the morning and eat meals at typical mealtimes.
- **Sleep associations:** These are objects, people, and environments the brain connects with sleep.
  - Night wakings are a normal part of the sleep cycle. Whatever your child needs to calm down and fall asleep at bedtime is what they need to get back to sleep easily during those normal night wakings.
  - **Tip:** The *what, where,* and *how* of falling asleep at bedtime should stay the same all night long.
  - **Tip:** If your child has a sleep association to a special thing like a blanket or stuffie, get multiples of that thing and rotate them.

Pillow Point

Whatever a person needs to calm down and fall asleep is what they need to return to sleep easily during night wakings, which are part of a normal sleep cycle.

Chapter 3

What Is Healthy Sleep for Neurodiverse Kids?

The moms of a three-year-old boy named Adam, who had speech and fine motor delays, once came to me in tears because their son wouldn't nap and wouldn't sleep for more than nine hours a night. The typical recommendation is for kids that age to sleep at least ten to twelve hours, and Adam's parents were worried a sleep deficiency might harm his development.

As they described his sleep routine to me, I was left awestruck and a little jealous. I wished I could be more like them. If there were an Olympic medal for bedtime routines, this was unquestionably gold. Each night at 7 p.m., the moms gave Adam a bath, rubbed him down with lavender lotion, put on organic cotton pajamas, brushed his teeth, had him use the toilet and wipe with bamboo toilet paper, and read him two books. Then they put Adam in his crib, turned on brown noise and a soft yellow nightlight (both programmed to stay on all night long), said their I-love-yous, turned out the light, and left the room.

Yet Adam wouldn't fall asleep for another one or two hours. He talked and sang to himself until about 9:30 p.m., when he finally conked out. Then he woke up like clockwork at 6:30 a.m. All in all, this wasn't a bad situation. But it wasn't the ideal. Adam was falling asleep later and sleeping fewer hours than recommended, and he didn't nap during the day. He would occasionally tolerate a one-hour quiet time in the crib, but he never fell asleep. This drove these very caring, conscientious parents nuts, since they wanted to do anything they could to maximize Adam's development. They wondered how he could be happy and not sleepy even though he rarely got the amount of sleep he was supposed to get. After our initial meeting, we tried starting his bedtime routine later, closer to the time he usually fell asleep. This was intended to limit the time he was awake in his crib, which is generally helpful. In Adam's case, it didn't help because he needed that hour-long wind-down time no matter what time he went to bed. If he went to bed later, he fell asleep later.

We also tried intermittent reminders, such as opening the door and saying, "It's bedtime, time for sleeping." Sometimes neurodiverse kids of any age need these reminders because they can get lost in their own worlds and forget that the task at hand is sleep. Beth, an older child I worked with, had a pattern of moving her arms and legs as if she were making snow angels while reciting monologues from Disney movies until she fell asleep. Her parents would pop in every fifteen to twenty minutes to remind her, "Calm body, quiet voice," and these reminders drastically shortened the time it took her to fall asleep. In Adam's case, the reminders interfered with his own self-soothing routine.

This became a situation where I shifted from the ideal to the real. When kids are neurodiverse, their real sleep might *be* their ideal sleep. I often work with families for whom there isn't a single thing I would change about their routines. Instead, I recommend adjusting expectations and keeping an eye on daytime mood and functioning. This is what these moms did, accepting that if Adam remained happy and energized during the day, then his nighttime sleep must be good enough for him.

I'm frequently asked what good sleep is. Is it ideal for a three-year-old to sleep ten to twelve hours, to have a bedtime of 7:30 to 8 p.m., or to take a nap only three days a week? Is it healthiest for toddlers to co-sleep or sleep independently? What is the best bedtime snack, nightlight color, or number of books to read? The answer to all those questions is, it depends. It varies based on your family structure and culture, on your child's age, schedule, and temperament, on the home environment and neighborhood, and on and on. If you throw neurodiversity into that mix, it's even tougher to nail down a definition of good sleep. By and large, guidelines for hours of sleep recommended for children aren't based on research showing what amount of sleep children *should* get.[1] They are based on surveys of how much sleep children *already get*. There are studies showing that at school age, getting less than ten hours of sleep per night is associated with lower grades, that a bedtime before 9 p.m. leads to better sleep, and that increasing sleep time by thirty minutes improves the skills children need to succeed in school. There are not studies demonstrating the exact number of hours a child should get at each age for ideal health and development. A benchmark I use is that a ten-year-old child should get about ten hours of sleep and have a bedtime before 9 p.m., but this is based on loose extrapolation from many studies in combination with my professional experience. There aren't studies demonstrating that ten hours of sleep is needed for optimal functioning of a ten-year-old child, let alone a ten-year-old child with ASD and ADHD. The American Academy of Sleep Medicine guidelines, listed in the sidebar below, are what most sleep experts use.

AMERICAN ACADEMY OF SLEEP MEDICINE RECOMMENDATIONS

Here are the American Academy of Sleep Medicine's recommended daily hours of sleep for children, from birth through age twelve.

- **Infant (4 to 12 months old):** 12–16 hours, including one to four naps
- **Toddler (1 to 2 years old):** 11–14 hours, including one nap (shift to one nap by around twelve to eighteen months)
- **Preschool (3 to 5 years old):** 10–13 hours, including possibly one nap (naps typically end between age three and five)
- **School age (6 to 12 years old):** 9–12 hours at night, no daytime sleep

How do sleep experts define healthy sleep?[2] In 2014, a renowned sleep physician, Daniel Buysse, published a paper asking, "What is sleep health and does it matter?"[3] He explored the idea that healthy sleep is more than not having a sleep disorder. For adults, he came up with the acronym *SATED* for what healthy sleep entails: *satisfaction* with sleep, *alertness* during the day, appropriate *timing* of sleep at night, *efficient* sleep (or being asleep most of the time you're in bed), and adequate total sleep *duration* of six to ten hours a day.

Adapting this to fit children and teens took three of the best sleep psychologist researchers in the world: Lisa Meltzer, Ariel Williamson, and Jodi Mindell.[4] Expanding on Dr. Buysse's work, they added a *B* for *behaviors* to make the acronym *B-SATED*. *Behaviors* refer to the things a child does at bedtime and as they're falling asleep. They also highlighted additional considerations for children:

- Especially during infancy, sleep needs are extremely variable. Some newborns sleep up to nineteen hours a day, and others might sleep nine hours a day. We all, of course, cross our fingers that we get the long sleeper, but unfortunately it's not up to us.

- The need for sleep during the day decreases at around kindergarten age, when most children no longer need a daytime nap.

- Most of what pediatric sleep experts know comes from what parents say, and parents can't know what is happening every minute their children are sleeping (or not sleeping).

For my own kids and for the families I work with in my practice, I loosely base my definition of healthy sleep on B-SATED:

B-SATED

Behaviors: Does your child have a consistent routine and sleep schedule? Do they fall asleep independently without conflict or negative sleep associations?

Satisfaction: How do you and your child feel about their sleep?

Alertness: Is your child able to participate in school and other daytime activities?

Timing: Do they sleep at night and not during the day?

Efficiency: Does your child spend most of the time they are in bed sleeping, or do they lie awake for hours?

Duration: Do they fall asleep at bedtime within about thirty minutes and wake in the morning on their own? Do they seem awake and alert during the day? Refer to the American Academy of Sleep Medicine or the American Academy of Pediatrics guidelines, but rely more on how your child functions during the day.

Evaluating Your Own Kid

Where does this general advice leave parents of neurodiverse kids? How do we know if we're doing it right? Henry generally sleeps from 9:30 p.m. to 7 a.m. Since he's now school age, that matches the American Academy of Sleep Medicine's recommended range for hours of sleep. Well, he's been in this range since he was about three years old, so even though nothing has changed, his sleep has "improved" according to the charts.

Also, about four times per month, Henry can't fall asleep until midnight or 2 a.m., wakes up for an hour or two during the night, or wakes for the day at 4 a.m. When Henry was younger, our family's sleep would be a mess for two to four days when he got a new toy or was intensely focused on something, like whether Jupiter has an atmosphere or what year each letter in the Cyrillic alphabet was created. Now when he has trouble falling asleep or staying asleep, he often sneaks out of bed and draws pictures of imaginary solar systems or builds futuristic vehicles with Legos. While being awake after bedtime isn't ideal, lying in bed awake for long periods can make things worse.

Just about every time Henry has one of these stretches, his dad asks me why it happened or what woke Henry up. He hypothesizes several likely and often true causes: that Henry ate too much sugar, didn't get enough exercise, maybe got worried that our house number changed when we moved, and a litany of other things that are somewhat within our control. I occasionally get frustrated with these conversations because even if our habits were absolute perfection, something about being neurodiverse tends to get in the way of falling asleep and returning to sleep easily. None of us can force sleep. We can only set up the right conditions and wait for sleep to arrive. During Henry's rougher sleep periods, I tell myself that, most of the time, he is still getting the sleep he needs to continue growing and developing.

If it's true that there is so much variability and subjectivity in healthy sleep, what guidelines should we follow, and how do we know we are making the best decisions for our child and family? Well, we look at our kids and how they are functioning. Ask yourself (and your child if possible) if they do the following:

- Sleep at night and not during the day, except for appropriate naps?
- Wake in the morning on their own or have to be dragged out of bed? Are they irritable upon waking?
- Fall asleep during therapies, activities, or at school?
- Complain about their sleep or about feeling tired during the day?
- Say or indicate that something bothers them in their body when trying to fall asleep?
- Lie in bed awake for hours?
- Have radically different daytime behavior if they have a great (or awful) night's sleep?

You are the expert on your child. You know and can evaluate them best. If your child's sleep patterns lead to pretty good functioning on most days, I'd say that is healthy sleep.

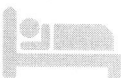

Tuck-In Tips

- Most sleep guidelines for kids are based on parent reports of how much sleep children are already getting.
- Healthy sleep might look different for someone who is neurodivergent.
- Use your child's daytime mood and functioning rather than number of hours to estimate sleep need.
- If you like acronyms, *B-SATED* is a good one to evaluate your child's sleep.

Pillow Point

The exact number of hours of sleep needed for optimum development is not known, so rely on your child's daytime alertness, behavior, and functioning to determine adequate sleep duration.

Chapter 4

Why Do Neurodiverse Kids Have So Many Sleep Problems?

One person whose shoulders I stand on is Dr. Beth Malow, a pediatric sleep pioneer and *the* sleep and neurodiversity expert. I may have written *this* book, but she has been there, done that, with her own book many years ago.[1] The first time I heard her speak, she was sharing her research on sleep and ASD with the Children's Hospital of Philadelphia. It was a great talk, and I wondered what had inspired her to dedicate her life's work to this little-known field. Near the end of her talk, she mentioned that she had children on the autism spectrum, and I thought, *OK, now I get it*. But honestly, I did not get it. I was galaxies away from understanding the complexities of neurodiverse parenting.

The second time I heard Dr. Malow speak was a few months after my son was diagnosed with ASD. I was raw with worry, protectiveness, confusion, worry, and more worry. I felt like I was drowning. The routine of working at the Sleep Center at Children's Hospital of Philadelphia and the satisfaction of helping other families barely kept my head above water. Dr. Malow talked about the very condition that would have such a profound influence on my family's future. I vacillated between wanting to tell her everything and wanting to run out of the room as she finished her last words. I chose the latter.

Well, nearly ten years later, she is still *the* sleep and neurodiversity expert, though now she has plenty of good company.

Dr. Malow has conducted a gazillion studies, written hundreds of articles, and given countless presentations highlighting how much, in what way, and why neurodiversity and sleep difficulties go hand in hand.[2]

Another true sleep pioneer is Dr. Jodi Mindell, my mentor, friend, and colleague and one of the people responsible for propelling the field of behavioral sleep medicine into existence. She divides sleep symptoms into three buckets: One bucket represents medical sleep problems, another bucket is behavioral sleep problems and habits, and the third bucket is overflowing with problems that aren't sleep disorders per se but can disrupt sleep (see "Sleep Buckets" illustration below). When I first meet families, I warn them that I ask about a *lot* of details. These details help me situate their family's sleep problems into one or more of these buckets.

Sleep Buckets

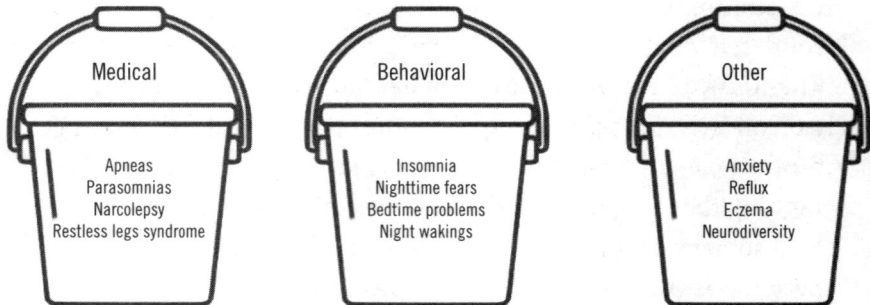

Medical	Behavioral	Other
Apneas	Insomnia	Anxiety
Parasomnias	Nighttime fears	Reflux
Narcolepsy	Bedtime problems	Eczema
Restless legs syndrome	Night wakings	Neurodiversity

The medical-sleep-problems bucket contains sleep disorders such as obstructive sleep apnea (OSA), and restless legs syndrome (RLS). Many parents hope their child's sleep problems are in the medical-sleep-problems bucket because that would mean (1) it's not their fault, since they didn't create this problem; (2) there is a clear explanation for these sleep difficulties; and (3) there must be a straightforward solution.

Here's the thing, and please hear me loud and clear: We all do the best we can in the face of a tough situation with a child we love dearly. We also all need sleep ourselves and aren't at our best when we are sleep-deprived. Regardless of what bucket the problem is in, the issue isn't faulty parenting. Even if someone is still rocking their fifty-five-pound child to sleep, or a child can only fall asleep rubbing a parent's nose, they are in this situation because their whole family needs sleep! Also, even if a child's sleep symptoms are due to a medical sleep problem, the solution isn't always straightforward.

The second bucket is behavioral sleep problems, and those include insomnia, nighttime fears, bedtime problems, and night wakings. Sloshing around in the last bucket are problems that aren't themselves sleep disorders but can still cause sleep disruptions. This one is a big, big bucket, and I want to start with something at the bottom of it: the underlying biological reasons why neurodivergent kids might have sleep problems.

Neurodiversity-Related Sleep Problems

This section was a doozy for me to write because there are many possible biological reasons why sleep problems are more common in neurodiverse kids, but there are not many definitive answers. New findings related to genetics, brain structures, and other physiological systems are published all the time, and someday this will lead to advances in the way we treat sleep problems in neurodiverse kids.[3] Here is what we know right now:

Genetics

The most likely reason for a child's neurodiversity *and* for their sleep problem is genetics.[4] ADHD, ASD, and other neurodevelopmental conditions are highly heritable, and so are many sleep problems. One explanation for this is that the same variations in a child's genome that caused neurodivergence might also cause sleep problems. Another explanation is that certain genetic variations are more common in people with neurodevelopmental conditions. For example, genes related to insomnia as well as genes related to circadian rhythm have already been identified, and variations in these genes are more common in people with ADHD, ASD, and other neurodiversities.

Sleep Pressure

In chapter 2, I talk about three ways that our bodies know to "turn on" sleep. The first is sleep pressure. Our bodies are always trying to get back to a steady, non-sleepy state, so the further we get from our last sleep period, the more we need to sleep. There is evidence that sleep pressure is not as strong in those with neurodevelopmental conditions, and/or that sleep pressure might be taken away more quickly. This would make it harder for a neurodiverse person to fall asleep in the first place, more likely to wake up too early, and prone to getting less sleep overall.[5] I can't tell you how many times I've heard families say that if their neurodiverse child takes even a ten-minute nap, their typical bedtime will be out the window. Or that their child's bedtime is 11:30 p.m. because if they fall asleep at 8 p.m., they are wide awake for the day at 3 a.m. Although I am a true believer in behavioral approaches, there is no incentive system, amount of ignoring, or other behavioral technique that can force the body to fall asleep or stay asleep if there isn't enough sleep pressure. On the flip side, behavioral approaches are very helpful for setting up the right conditions for sleep, which includes safely, calmly, and quietly staying in bed. I discuss this more in part 2.

Circadian System

The second way the body knows to turn on sleep is from an internally generated biological pattern that repeats on its own every twenty-four hours, the circadian rhythm. The two most important influences on the circadian rhythm are morning light exposure and the timing of meals. There are multiple differences in the circadian system that can affect sleep, even if the symptoms look the same. Studies have shown that children with ADHD tend to be night owls, and they may have a later circadian rhythm, leading to trouble falling asleep. While their circadian rhythm may be set later than ideal, the clock itself works just fine. This is different from ASD, where the clock isn't necessarily always running behind, but it is inconsistent from night to night. One night the circadian clock might say, "It's three in the morning and time to sleep," while another night the message might be, "It's three in the morning and time to wake up."

Another potential hiccup in the circadian system is how the body responds to light. Sunlight influences our circadian clock by traveling from the eye to the suprachiasmatic nucleus (SCN) in the brain, which is the conductor of our internal circadian rhythm.[6] Once the SCN gets the signal from the eye's retina, it sends the messages to other parts of the brain that control hunger, thirst, body temperature, neurotransmitters, and hormones. In the case of sleep, the SCN signals the pineal gland to release melatonin, the hormone that causes us to feel sleepy, fall asleep, and stay asleep. There can be a problem with any part of this system, starting with the eye, if a person is visually impaired and can't perceive light, and including the pineal gland (and the release of melatonin). Even if a child has 20/20 vision, the way the SCN responds to light might be altered in neurodiverse kids.

While melatonin is certainly related to sleep difficulties in neurodiverse children, we don't know precisely how. The circadian system could be working perfectly, but the amount of melatonin released might not be enough to turn on sleep, or it might not be released long enough or fast enough. In children with ADHD, no consistent melatonin dysfunction has been found. In those with ASD, multiple alterations in melatonin could explain frequent, long, middle-of-the-night wakings or unpredictable sleep schedules. Alterations in neurotransmitters linked to waking, such as serotonin and orexin, may also play a role in nighttime sleep problems.[7]

Despite the circadian clock being internally generated, a wayward circadian rhythm can be helped with behavioral treatment. For example, one treatment for the too-late circadian rhythm common in ADHD involves morning exposure to sunlight or to a special light that mimics sunlight. This can nudge the rhythm earlier, reduce daytime sleepiness, and shorten the time it takes to fall asleep at night.[8]

Turning Off Wakefulness

While we know that our circadian clock and sleep pressure turn sleep on, the systems that turn wakefulness off are a different story. Contrary to what we might assume, sleep and wake aren't opposite ends of a spectrum; they are completely different processes. In chapter 12, I discuss *how* to turn wakefulness off; here I explain *why* this could be harder in neurodiverse children and teens.

Stress Response System

The hypothalamic pituitary axis and the autonomic nervous system are responsible for how our bodies respond to stress.[9] These systems are activated by any cause of stress, from being chased by a tiger to starting a new middle school, from sensitivity to sound to greeting a teacher. The hormone triggered by stress, cortisol, is also the wake-up hormone, and it is triggered when melatonin turns off. While the amount of cortisol in a neurodiverse person might not be any different than in a neurotypical person, the fluctuations in cortisol are much greater.[10] Sometimes neurodivergent people show a blunted stress response to situations that a neurotypical person might be freaking out about, while in other situations, a neurodiverse person might have an extreme stress response to something that isn't typically considered stressful. These fluctuations in cortisol can interfere with effectively turning off wakefulness.

Internal Communication

Another part of the brain that can interfere with turning off wakefulness is the default mode network (DMN). The DMN is the state of the brain's internal communication system when it's not engaged in an activity. It is a resting state, a baseline.[11] Despite not being involved in an externally stimulating task, parts of the brain are still active at rest and while sleeping. The DMN is still working (though it ought to be taking it easy). During sleep, the DMN should reduce communication specifically between two parts of the brain, the thalamus (the hub of sensory information) and the prefrontal cortex (the information processing/thinking part of the brain).[12] The thalamus sends sensory signals to different parts of the cortex where the information is processed. For example, sounds are sent from the ear to the thalamus, and then the thalamus sends the signal to the auditory cortex, where the sound is processed and interpreted. The thalamus is also responsible for sleep, attention, and alertness.

In children with ASD, there can be too much communication between the thalamus and the cortex, and this can lead to difficulties in sensory processing, which also interfere with sleep. Our senses shouldn't be as active during sleep as they are when we are awake. A colleague of mine studied this in preschoolers with ASD and found that even though the children were sleeping, the auditory cortex was still activated. This suggests the thalamus was still sending sensory input to the cortex during sleep,[13] which would theoretically make it difficult to turn off wakefulness. Difficulty sleeping in neurodiverse kids may relate to differences in the DMN itself and/or to communication problems between areas of the brain related to sleep and wake, such as the thalamus and the prefrontal cortex.

Glymphatic System

Another brain process that is not as well understood when it comes to neurodiversity and sleep is the glymphatic system — correct, this is not the lymphatic system. The glymphatic system is responsible for getting rid of the neurotoxic waste produced by the central nervous system when we are awake.[14] Importantly, it is only turned on during sleep. Early research shows that this sleep-dependent cleanup system may be altered in children with ADHD and/or ASD, and it may also be different in adults with insomnia.[15] In addition to the possibility that an altered glymphatic system causes sleep problems, it is also possible that poor sleep causes problems with the glymphatic system.

Sleep is more complicated than most people think. A lot goes on in the brain while we're in slumberland. When there are problems with underlying biological processes, sleep suffers. And when the stress response, communication, or cleanup systems aren't working as intended, turning off wakefulness is more difficult.

The Reverse: Do Sleep Problems Cause Neurodivergence?

If sleep problems in neurodiverse kids are caused by differences in underlying sleep processes, what about the reverse? Is it possible that poor sleep and differences in sleep processes cause neurodivergence?

In a word, no.

Poor sleep can sometimes be an early indicator of a neurodevelopmental condition.[16] A late circadian rhythm and insufficient sleep might cause decreased attention, lack of focus, and increased hyperactivity. The symptoms of insufficient sleep can look a lot like mild ADHD; however, poor sleep on its own does not *cause* the full constellation of ADHD symptoms. Not getting sufficient sleep might lead to more stimming or decreased social interactions, but sleep deprivation doesn't *cause* ASD. If you are concerned that your child might have ADHD or ASD, or if something just seems off, it's a good idea to prioritize sleep. However, don't wait for perfect sleep before seeking help. It's awful to wait six months for a sleep appointment and then another four months to work on the sleep problem, only to be told a child needs a developmental evaluation, and the wait is another year. Schedule appointments or get on waitlists while you're working to improve your child's sleep. If sleep gets better and your concerns go away, you can always cancel.

This is a lot of information. To summarize, there are a boatload of underlying biological reasons why neurodivergent children and teens might have more sleep problems. In addition to biological factors, there are also medical and behavioral sleep disorders, co-occurring medical and psychological conditions, and rare diseases that relate to neurodivergence and have such a big impact on sleep that they each get their own chapter! Stay tuned.

Tuck-In Tips

- There is an increased risk of sleep problems in neurodiverse children and teens, and genetics are likely a major cause of both poor sleep and neurodiversity.
- In neurodivergent people, differences in the biological mechanisms underlying sleep (circadian rhythm, sleep pressure) may interfere with sleep.
- Alterations in the brain's stress response, communication, and neurotoxin removal systems also cause problems for turning off wakefulness.
- Poor sleep does not cause neurodivergence.

Pillow Point

There are multiple biological differences in neurodiverse kids that increase the risk of sleep problems.

Chapter 5

Is It a Medical Sleep Disorder?

Medical sleep disorders are rare in the general population of children who don't have neurodevelopmental or medical conditions. For example, the prevalence of obstructive sleep apnea (OSA; pauses in breathing during sleep due to the collapse of the airway) is 2 to 5 percent; periodic limb movement disorder (PLMD; limb movements during sleep that wake up the brain) is 0.3 percent; and narcolepsy (a neurological condition leading to sleepiness and difficulty regulating sleep/wake cycles) is 0.013 to 0.025 percent. I have been lucky enough to work at large children's hospitals with sleep programs, so I've seen hundreds of children and teens with rare sleep conditions.

When I was in the last year of my doctoral program, I saw a twelve-year-old boy named Max who changed my whole perspective on sleep and mental health. He was brought to the clinic because he was sleepy. He had newly diagnosed ADHD but was not taking medications yet. He had (and was still having) extensive orthodontic treatment because, at times, his jaw hung open and he felt like he couldn't control it. His mom thought he just wasn't paying attention and that, essentially, Max was kind of out of it. He had become socially withdrawn and was falling asleep a lot during the day and early evening, preventing him from participating in sports, riding his bike, and going to birthday parties. Max was also falling asleep multiple times per day at school. His mom showed me copies of the multiple emails teachers had sent her. At first they mostly complained about Max sleeping during class, and then they reflected increasing concern. His homeroom teacher had been teaching for thirty years, and she said she hadn't seen anything like this before. Max had also gained weight over the past year, which the family attributed to him being less active and less involved with friends.

In the clinic, trainees like me usually saw a new family first to get the scoop. Then the physician, the supervising psychologist, and I would go to a conference room to talk about potential diagnoses, additional tests that were needed, possible first steps for treatment, and recommendations to discuss with the family. Being a psychology trainee, I interviewed Max and his mother, and I immediately jumped to the conclusion that depression and untreated ADHD were the culprits. I wanted to get this kid some therapy immediately! I reported the symptoms to the excellent physician and psychologist I worked with, and we went back into the room to talk more with the family. I was surprised that the physician ordered an overnight sleep study with a daytime nap study to further evaluate Max's sleepiness. For the sleep study to be accurate, he couldn't be on any antidepressants or medications for ADHD because they can interfere with the results. Because our sleep lab had a waitlist and his appointment was three months later, Max wouldn't be able to start any medications until after the study.

After work, I complained to my fellow trainees. I thought it was a waste to put him through an unnecessary sleep study when, really, he just needed help for his depression and ADHD. In my mind, he needed a great therapist, potentially an antidepressant and/or medication for his ADHD, physical activity, and some fun experiences with peers. Max tugged at my heartstrings, and I badly wanted him to get some relief. After he had the sleep study, I waited days and days for the results, eager to get the ball rolling on the treatment of his depression and ADHD.

Welp, I couldn't believe it. His sleep study clearly showed that he had narcolepsy, an incredibly rare sleep disorder that explained his various symptoms. Max's mouth hung open intermittently during the day after all that orthodontia because of cataplexy. Cataplexy is the loss of muscle tone with strong emotion. This can happen to people with narcolepsy when they are surprised or angry or they hear something funny or scary. Sometimes the person falls to the ground, but other times it is more subtle, and it might be a slack jaw, wobbly knees, or a floppy hand that drops a pencil. Weight gain is also common in people with narcolepsy. And of course, he was depressed and withdrawn! Living with this undiagnosed sleep disorder for years while becoming increasingly sleepy and isolated led to his depression, not the other way around. I was humbled, to say the least.

I saw this family six months later, after Max had been taking medication for his narcolepsy (which also treated his ADHD) and was consistently sleeping on the schedule we had prescribed, which included planned naps. While he was still sleepy at the end of the day, the change was astounding. He was beaming. He reported that he had tried out for baseball, was frequently riding his bike to the park with friends, had weekly therapy, and was mostly staying awake in school. Imagine that — Max was understood, validated, correctly diagnosed, and appropriately treated. Of course, every sleep problem isn't a medical sleep disorder, but it's critical to take a good look at that bucket.

The Necessary Weirdness of Sleep Studies

For medical sleep problems, including sleep apnea, periodic limb movement disorder, restless sleep disorder, and narcolepsy, an overnight sleep study called a polysomnogram (PSG) in a sleep lab is needed to make a diagnosis. Whenever I describe a PSG to families, they tend to look at me as if I have three heads. It's a strange overnight experience that, as of this writing, must be conducted in a lab, and most parents want to know how the heck their family will make it through to the morning. I understand the skepticism. Most of the time, the experience isn't nearly as rough as people think, especially if they go to a pediatric sleep lab. Unfortunately, pediatric sleep labs are not everywhere, but a lab that studies both adults and children will be fine, too. To find a lab near you, check the resources section at the end of this book.

What happens during a PSG? Typically, a parent and child arrive at the sleep lab in the early evening with the child's favorite pj's, snacks, books, pillow, stuffies, and usual medications. The child is then prepared for an overnight electroencephalogram (EEG), which involves placing sticky EEG leads on the scalp in specific places, to measure the brain waves. The child's head is often wrapped up in a turban to cover the whole shebang. Other sticky sensors are placed near the eyes and on the jaw and legs to measure movements during the sleep stages. The sleep technologist also attaches stretchy bands around the chest and belly, a nasal cannula (short nose tubes) just outside the nose, a pulse oximeter on a finger or toe, and a microphone to hear snoring. Nothing involves pain, but it is unquestionably weird.

Overnight, a video also records the child, who sleeps in their own hospital crib or bed. The parent stays in the room but has to sleep in a separate bed, so their own breathing and movements don't interfere with the child's results. As needed throughout the night, the sleep technologist will come in to adjust the wires, stickers, and belts on the child. The study is completed by early morning, and then participants can go home. The only lingering issue is having to wash the sticky stuff from the EEG leads out of the child's hair!

To evaluate daytime sleepiness, the day after the PSG, children sometimes also have a daytime nap study called a multiple sleep latency test. In that case, parent and child hang out in the lab the following day, and the child is given the chance to take four or five twenty-minute naps. For the nap study, breathing isn't usually measured, since it was studied the previous night. Once all the testing is done, it takes a sleep doctor one to two weeks to interpret the study, which requires analyzing data from the whole night in thirty-second increments.

Parents usually worry about how their child will react to all this, but kids are typically OK. Experienced sleep technicians have seen every type of situation you can think of, and they almost always get the data they need. Parents are usually the ones suffering in the morning from having to sleep in the uncomfortable, convertible chair-bed that labs usually provide.

If a sleep doctor prescribes an overnight sleep study for your child, always ask the clinic staff or the sleep lab for some extra EEG leads and a nasal cannula, so you can practice ahead of time at home and acclimate your child to the experience. Place the circular EEG stickers (with strings attached to simulate the wires, if you want) in a few places on the scalp using Scotch tape or painter's tape. You can rub each spot on the scalp with a grainy facial scrub; this is very similar to the stuff technicians use to prepare the scalp underneath the EEG stickers (the whole scalp isn't scrubbed, just where EEG leads are placed). You might also search online for pictures, videos, and stories others have posted. Since most pediatric sleep labs have long wait times for appointments, you will likely have weeks to prepare your child. That said, don't worry too much about the study. For parents of neurodiverse kids, an overnight sleep study isn't fun, but it isn't always more challenging than whatever they already go through.

Many parents ask why their child can't do the sleep study at home, which would be much easier for everyone. While home sleep apnea tests (HSATs) are available for adults, as of this writing, these are not yet an option for children outside of research studies. One reason is that most HSAT devices only test for sleep-disordered breathing. Most don't measure brain waves or limb movements, and they don't screen for seizures or analyze sleep stages. The second reason is that children move around *a lot* in their sleep, and the wonderful sleep techs need to adjust the sensors and equipment throughout the night. One day pediatric sleep tests might be routinely conducted at home, but not yet.

Apneas

Apneas are temporary pauses in breathing that cause oxygen levels to drop. This triggers a survival reflex, also called fight-or-flight mode. Our heart rate and blood pressure go up, adrenaline is released, and we wake up to inhale oxygen. While many people have no idea they've woken up, others wake coughing or gasping. Other symptoms include mouth breathing and/or waking in the morning with a headache. With young kids, it can sometimes induce a new onset of bed-wetting after being potty trained for several months. Apneas can cause sleepiness, increases in behavior problems, decreases in neurocognitive functioning, and overall poor quality of life even when people get enough hours of sleep. Poor sleep quality due to apnea usually leads to feeling unrefreshed regardless of sleep duration.

There are two types of apneas. Obstructive sleep apnea (OSA) is the most common. This happens when the airway is fully or partially blocked, causing restricted breathing and a drop in oxygen. Fight-or-flight mode is activated, leading to waking up multiple times throughout the night. There is a common misunderstanding that snoring is a sign of a good, deep sleep, but it is actually the main symptom of OSA. Any child with snoring (other than when sick) should be screened for OSA. Recognizing when snoring is only snoring versus obstructive sleep apnea is impossible without a PSG.[1]

OSA is most common in children ages two to eight, since that is when tonsils and adenoids are biggest and the airway is still small, leading to a crowded space. Other risk factors for OSA include low muscle tone (present in many neurodiverse kids), obesity, and/or a small jaw or a lower jaw that is set back, as with an overbite. Another risk factor is the way soft tissue is distributed around the face, as with Down syndrome. Almost all rare genetic and craniofacial conditions come with a higher risk of OSA. For example, the risk of OSA in the general population is from 2 to 5 percent, and the risk of OSA in people with Down syndrome is as high as 75 percent. In general, OSA worsens during REM because of our paralyzed, floppy muscles. Positional OSA (POSA) is ob-structive sleep apnea that only occurs when sleeping in a certain position (usually on the back).[2] POSA is more common in adults (55 percent) than in children (18.7 percent), and children with POSA are more likely to be older, be obese, have small tonsils, and have less-severe OSA.

If the sleep study shows that your child has OSA, what's next? You'll likely be told to make an appointment with a pediatric oto-laryngologist — or ear, nose, and throat doctor — to talk about surgically removing the tonsils and adenoids (an adenotonsillec-tomy). While surgery is no trip to Disneyland, adenotonsillectomy cures OSA in most children.[3] Surgery may be less successful in older adolescents, obese children and teens, those with low mus-cle tone, and those with craniofacial differences. Aside from ade-notonsillectomy, there are multiple other surgical and nonsurgical options.[4]

Positive airway pressure (PAP) is the next line of treatment. A PAP mask looks like an oxygen mask and is connected to a tube that is connected to a machine about the size of a lunchbox. The machine blows air through the tube and the mask to keep the air-way open during sleep. CPAP (continuous positive airway pres-sure) provides continuous pressure during the inhale and exhale. BPAP (bilevel PAP) provides one pressure on the inhale and a lower pressure on the exhale. This lower pressure makes it easier for the body to get rid of excess carbon dioxide, for example, if a child has a musculoskeletal condition where it's harder to exhale effectively.

It's important to acknowledge that getting used to PAP can be difficult for anyone, regardless of age,[5] and it is often a gradual process lasting weeks or months. In general, helping a child get used to PAP (called desensitization) starts with exploring or play-ing with the equipment and putting it on other people or stuffed animals. The next step is to get used to wearing the mask without the air. This step-by-step work continues until the person can fall asleep with the PAP on and sleep with it on throughout the night. Wearing PAP consistently over weeks and months often requires significant reinforcement. At the clinic where I worked, our PAP team would sing a special song, give a patient a PAP trophy, and with their permission, put their photo on the PAP wall of champions.

Daysha, a sixteen-year-old with Williams syndrome, was one of my favorite patients ever. She had severe obstructive sleep apnea that persisted even after having her tonsils and adenoids removed. She was prescribed CPAP, and it was my job to help desensitize Daysha to the CPAP device, so that eventually she could wear it all night long. Her team knew it was important that she start wearing it ASAP. Armed with a plan and a mission, I walked purposefully into Daysha's room and was greeted with an enthusiastic welcome.

"Oh hey girl!" she said. "Do you like spaghetti?"

I quickly shifted gears. Instead of CPAP, we talked about our favorite pasta shapes, meatballs, a recent shopping trip, and her upcoming sleepover with friends. When I tried to steer us back to CPAP, Daysha let me know that no-way, no-how was she going to wear that thing. She rolled her eyes and in her cool teenage way told me about her new shoes and how she liked to collect old jewelry from thrift stores.

"You know me and my girls," she said. "We go into the Goodwill, and we are not shy. We go right up to the counter and tell that old lady to bring out the best bling. I love that bling. I like the bling stickers from Michael's, too, and I even blinged out my pencil case. See?" She proudly showed me the case covered in small pink and gold gem heart stickers.

I jumped right on that bling bandwagon and suggested we bling out her CPAP machine. In an unbelievable coincidence, I had some gem stickers that I had bought weeks earlier for my son's school project. They were in my bag because we hadn't used them, and I was planning to return them on my way home from work. Daysha loved the stickers but remained wary of the CPAP.

"Girl," she told me, "I do not want to bring that ugly mess to my Friday sleepovers! It will look so dumb to my crew."

We went back and forth, weaving talk about Daysha's favorite clothes, shows, and celebrities with snippets of CPAP talk. Eventually, we agreed on a plan where she would practice wearing her CPAP daily while watching reruns of the baking show *Nailed It!* Every time she practiced for at least fifteen minutes, Daysha got one row of five bling stickers. If she put it on and fell asleep with it at bedtime, she got five rows of bling. Once she could fall asleep with it and wear it all night for ten nights, Daysha would earn the motherload of gem stickers: an entire package. As a compromise, I told her that if she wore it the other nights of the week, she did not have to bring her CPAP to her Friday sleepovers. Lucky for me, this approach worked!

Adenotonsillectomy and PAP are the most researched treatments in pediatric OSA, and those are the treatments that should be tried first. If neither surgery nor PAP are possible or effective, discuss other options with your child's sleep physician, ENT doctor, neurologist, pulmonologist, or other medical provider.[6]

Some potential alternative options include high-flow oxygen, which is delivered by the same type of nasal cannula a child wears during a sleep study. It can be effective at preventing drops in oxygen, but it is not as good as PAP for reducing heart rate or the cardiac stress due to the fight-or-flight response.[7] Certain medications might also help. Nasal steroid sprays (like fluticasone) or allergy medicines (like montelukast) may shrink the adenoids and/or tonsils, which can decrease OSA symptoms, but they may not take away OSA entirely.[8] There is a new medication (combining oxybutynin and atomoxetine)[9] that has demonstrated promising results in adults, but as of this writing, it is only available in the context of a research study. Similarly, weight-loss medications are used to treat obesity-related OSA in adults, but these medications are not yet available for children. These medications could be game changers for OSA treatment.

There are multiple orthodontic devices and procedures that can increase the size of the airway and decrease OSA.[10] These include mandibular advancement surgery, rapid maxillary expansion, and orthodontic appliances that may or may not be removable. For a child or teen with a large tongue or another craniofacial condition that increases the likelihood of OSA, there are other surgical approaches, such as tongue-reduction surgery, that aim to make the airway less crowded.[11] A newer treatment called hypoglossal nerve stimulation requires surgery to implant a device near the clavicle that stimulates the airway muscles to stay active even during sleep. However, as of this writing, it is only available to children and teens in the context of a research study.

Positional therapy is used to treat POSA, which is when OSA occurs only when sleeping in a certain position. There are pajama shirts with Velcro strips or pockets on the back for tennis balls, belts with foam wedges, and other clever ways to prevent sleeping in the position where OSA usually occurs, often on the back. Because children move around quite a bit during sleep, these positional methods are hard to keep in place, and thus they may be less effective.

Orofacial myofunctional therapy (OMT)[12] is typically administered by a speech pathologist, occupational therapist, or dental provider. OMT exercises strengthen muscles of the tongue, cheeks, uvula/soft palate, lips, and jaw.[13] OMT trains the tongue to rest in a position that doesn't block the airway and promotes nasal breathing (versus mouth breathing). Just like a body workout, the exercises must be practiced consistently to see improvement. My favorite OMT treatment for OSA is playing the didgeridoo, which is a musical instrument from indigenous Australia that makes a vibrating, droning sound. Playing the didgeridoo requires a special technique called circular breathing, and consistent practice has been shown to reduce the severity of OSA in adults. It has not yet been studied in children, but I'm looking forward to the day when it is![14]

For an overview of options, see table 5.1.

Table 5.1: Potential Treatments for OSA in Children and Teens

Treatment	What it is	Pros	Cons
Adenotonsil-lectomy	Surgery removing tonsils and adenoids	High success rate, doesn't require motivation, organization, or daily planning	Risk of surgery, not as effective for people with obesity, low tone, or craniofacial differences
CPAP or BPAP	Continuous air via a mask to hold open the airway during sleep	Good at reducing OSA when used appropriately	Often difficult to get used to, machine requires cleaning
High-flow nasal cannula	Oxygen via tubes right under the nose	Possibly easier to get used to than PAP, keeps oxygen levels from dropping	Does not prevent stress on the heart, still uncomfortable
Nasal steroids or antihista-mines	Nose spray or oral medication to shrink tonsils and adenoids	Fairly easy treatment, though kids often resist things up their noses (except for their own fingers)	May only help if OSA is mild and due to inflammation
Atomoxetine and oxybutynin	May improve upper airway muscle tone during sleep	Easy treatment, promising results in adults, atomoxetine alone has been widely studied in children for ADHD	Only available for children in research studies

Table 5.1: Potential Treatments for OSA in Children and Teens
(continued)

Treatment	What it is	Pros	Cons
Tongue reduction, other facial surgeries	Surgery to reduce tongue size or increase the size of the airway	Targeted to a specific problem or area, doesn't require motivation, organization, or daily planning	Only effective for certain conditions
Hypoglossal nerve stimulation	Implanted device that keeps airway muscles active during sleep	Doesn't require motivation, organization, or daily planning	Only available for children in research studies
Orthodontic procedures and devices	Surgery or appliance to move jaw forward and/or widen the soft palate	Effective for a specific problem or area	Only effective if OSA is due to jaw position or crowded airway
Positional therapy	Clothing, pillow, or other device that prevents sleeping in OSA-prone position (usually on back)	Easy to use, noninvasive	Only works in POSA, less effective with children, hard to keep in place
Orofacial myofunctional therapy	Exercises to strengthen tongue, cheeks, lips, jaw, and soft palate	Noninvasive	Only studied in adults, need specialized provider

The second type of apnea is central apnea, where the brain forgets to tell the body to take a breath. In premature infants, this is called apnea of prematurity (AOP), and the younger and smaller the infant, the more likely they are to have AOP. AOP is treated with medications such as caffeine and devices (such as PAP), and the apnea typically resolves as the infant gets bigger and stronger. Central apnea can also be caused by neuromuscular conditions, such as muscular dystrophy; by medical conditions that affect the heart, brain stem, or spinal cord; by structural malformations, such as Chiari malformations or brain tumors; by brain injuries from stroke or trauma; and by medications, such as opioids. Once the reason for the central apnea has been identified and addressed, treatment of central apnea is typically surgery or PAP.

Parasomnias

Parasomnias are a group of unusual behaviors during sleep that happen when wake behavior (such as talking, crying, or walking) intrudes into sleep. This mostly occurs during non-REM (NREM) sleep. In essence, during NREM parasomnias, the person is asleep but acting as if they are awake. Even knowing the person is asleep, it can be strange at best and scary at worst to see a child in one of these episodes. Parasomnias often have a genetic basis, and if your child has them, there's a good chance that someone in your family had them, too. Many kids experience parasomnias as a normal part of growing up, and most kids grow out of them by late school age. Parasomnias typically happen in the first third of the night, when there is the most NREM sleep. People usually have no idea they've had a parasomnia.

Confusional Arousals, Sleep Terrors, and Sleepwalking

NREM parasomnias include confusional arousals, sleep terrors, and sleepwalking. Confusional arousals are brief disturbances in sleep where the child might sit up or call out and then go back to sleep within a few minutes. Sleep terrors are more intense. Sometimes known as night terrors, they also happen during naps. About 30 percent of children experience sleep terrors. They happen as early as nine months and are most common between ages three and seven. Sleep terrors often begin with an alarming scream or cry; the child seems frightened or panicked and can be inconsolable. There may also be increased heart rate and breathing, sweating, and dilated pupils. It's hard to believe that something so shocking isn't terrifying for your child, but they truly are fast asleep and not having a horrible dream. Even though I know this, the one time my son had a sleep terror, I ran to his room faster than I've ever run, picked him up out of his crib, and repeatedly called his name. He was confused and looked like he just woke up, which actually he had!

Sleepwalking is an NREM parasomnia that requires attention to safety. People who sleepwalk can engage in familiar behaviors, and I've seen more kids than I can count who have peed in the closet, the trash can, or somewhere other than the toilet during a sleepwalking episode. I've seen multiple teenagers who have jumped out of windows while sleepwalking. During an episode, people can open doors, walk downstairs, or do other simple, familiar tasks. If your child experiences sleepwalking, make sure doors and windows are not easily opened, and they should be alarmed, if possible. Portable alarms on doors and windows are a good idea if your child sleepwalks and is in a different place, such as a hotel. Also move toys, bulky furniture, or anything that might be in their path when they get out of bed.

What should you do about confusional arousals, sleep terrors, and sleepwalking? First, keep in mind that your child will most likely grow out of these NREM parasomnias. Second, make sure they are getting enough sleep. The frequency of parasomnias is reduced with even thirty more minutes of sleep per night. Third, during the event itself, interact with your child as little as possible. Avoid saying your child's name, as they will wake more easily, which will only disrupt their sleep and can lead to more parasomnias. Stand in the doorway or near the bed quietly to see if they recognize you. If they are crying, asking to sleep in your bed, reaching for you, making sense, and clearly awake, it's not a parasomnia.

Some children experience parasomnias at about the same time every night. To break the cycle, parents can wake them just before a typical episode for several weeks. For example, if a child has a sleep terror most nights at 11:30 p.m., a parent could wake them at about 11 p.m. and make sure they are fully awake by taking them to the bathroom or having them take a drink of water. This puts them in a different stage of sleep that bypasses the parasomnia. These scheduled awakenings can be an absolute pain for a parent who is already sleep-deprived, which is why I can count on two hands the times I've recommended it.

Another potential treatment for NREM parasomnias, which is used more often in Europe than the United States, is 5-HTP (5-hydroxytryptophan) dietary supplements.[15] 5-HTP is a precursor to serotonin, which is a precursor to melatonin, and so theoretically it should impact sleep. In small European studies, 5-HTP was given shortly before bedtime for three weeks, and results were promising in terms of reducing sleep terrors. As with all supplements in the US, we don't know how much 5-HTP a given tablet or capsule contains, regardless of what the label says. Because there's no standard dosing or timing, we don't have clear guidance about when or how much to give.

Nightmare Disorder

Nightmare disorder is the most common REM-related parasomnia in children and teens. Nightmares are frightening dreams, often about survival, that cause sudden wakings. Unlike sleep terrors or sleepwalking, nightmares generally happen closer to the morning hours when the amount of REM sleep (dreaming sleep) is the highest. Nightmares typically start at three to six years old, reach their peak at six to ten years old, and decrease after age ten, though they never completely go away. Like parasomnias, nightmares tend to run in families. They are also influenced by psychological conditions, such as post-traumatic stress disorder or anxiety disorders, as well as by medications, such as antihistamines, beta blockers, antidepressants, and possibly melatonin. Nightmare *disorder* involves repeated nightmares that happen at least once per week for a prolonged period and are generally well remembered.

Research on nightmares in neurodiverse children and teens is all over the place.[16] Some studies have found increased nightmares in children with ADHD; however, it isn't clear that there are more nightmares associated with neurodevelopmental conditions in general. Results are difficult to interpret for a few reasons: (1) We don't know if neurodiverse kids have more nightmares or if they remember nightmares more than others due to lighter sleep and more wakings. (2) We can't know the content of someone else's nightmare directly. The child must tell us, write it down, or draw it, and this may not be possible. (3) The child must remember they even had a nightmare in the first place.

Research on treating nightmare disorder in children is sparse, and most studies to date haven't included neurodiversity as a factor. Imagery rehearsal therapy is one treatment for nightmares that are specific and repetitive.[17] This involves talking, drawing, and writing about the dream in detail, and then making a new script that changes the dream to be less frightening. The child might add silly elements to their dream, such as the monster having purple polka dots and a tutu. The child may add a helper who comes into the dream to protect them, or they may change the end of the dream so that they are safe and happy. Imagery rehearsal therapy should only be attempted with an experienced, licensed therapist or psychologist. A newer, promising treatment for both traumatic and nontraumatic nightmares is cognitive behavioral therapy for childhood nightmares.[18] This five-session treatment can be delivered in-person or virtually, and it involves relaxation strategies, sleep hygiene, and repeated exposure to the nightmare by talking and/or drawing about it. The child and the therapist create and practice a new version of the nightmare that has a more positive outcome.

Sleep-Related Rhythmic Movement Disorder (SRMD)

Most movements during sleep are normal and don't interfere with sleep, cause injury, or lead to daytime impairment. For example, hypnic jerks, sleep starts, and sleep myoclonus are quick movements or twitches that appear disruptive to sleep but are not. Sleep-related rhythmic movement disorder (SRMD) is more common in neurodiverse children and thought to be soothing due to vestibular stimulation. The vestibular system in the inner ear aids in sensing balance, movement, and the location of our bodies in space. Activation of the vestibular system, particularly repeated back and forth movements such as swinging or rocking, can bring on a feeling of calm and regulate neurotransmitters like serotonin that impact mood. Head banging and body rocking (with or without vocalizing) may be soothing, but they can also be so loud and intense that they wake others in the house or cause injury. It is difficult to teach a child to stop head banging and body rocking. We can introduce a replacement behavior, but that isn't always successful because SRMD occurs during a typical sleep cycle, and it is difficult to learn a new behavior when asleep. If your child or teen has been injured during sleep, talk to their pediatrician about options and move the bed away from walls so your child can't connect with a hard surface.

While most sleep movements are benign, sleep-related epilepsy is a rare disorder that requires treatment. If you suspect your child may be having seizures at night (they repeat the same movements, lose bowel or bladder control, or are injured), video the episodes if possible, and schedule an urgent visit to your child's pediatrician or neurologist.

Sleep Enuresis (Bed-Wetting)

Bed-wetting is only considered a sleep disorder in children older than five who wet the bed at least three times per week for more than three months. About 20 percent of five-year-olds still wet the bed at night. Sleep enuresis is more common in children with neurodevelopmental conditions, such as ADHD and ASD. This may be related to a decreased response to a full bladder or to an increased response to a bladder that is not completely empty or to constipation. Bed-wetting can also be caused by delays in the bladder's ability to hold urine overnight or to sleep disorders that fragment sleep, such as obstructive sleep apnea or periodic limb movement disorder.

Treatments for enuresis include bed-wetting alarms for the underwear that are triggered by a tiny amount of urine. Theoretically, the child will wake and go to the toilet before a full bed-wetting episode occurs. These alarms often disrupt everyone's sleep, which can be challenging for the whole household, and it can take several months to see an improvement. There are also medications that can reduce bed-wetting. These can be especially helpful in short-term situations like sleepovers.

Restless Sleep Disorders

Restless sleep disorders include periodic limb movement disorder (PLMD), restless legs syndrome (RLS), and restless sleep disorder (RSD). PLMD is characterized by small movements — such as flexing the big toe, ankle, and knee — that happen during sleep and wake up the brain. PLMD and RSD can only be diagnosed with an overnight sleep study. Up to 64 percent of children and teens with ADHD have PLMD, which leads to fragmented, poor-quality sleep and daytime sleepiness. Conversely, up to 91 percent of children and teens with PLMD have ADHD. Not only does ADHD itself relate to PLMD, but medications used to treat comorbid anxiety or depression (such as SSRIs and SNRIs) can increase these movements. Kids with both ADHD *and* PLMD are at increased risk of anxiety and more severe executive-function deficits.

While the symptoms of restless sleep disorder are not new, RSD only became an official sleep disorder in 2020. The criteria for a diagnosis are at least five large body movements (not just the legs) per hour during sleep, at least three times a week for three months. The movements must be documented by a sleep study and cause daytime impairment. Like OSA and PLMD, restless sleep disorder leads to sleep disruption, and as a result, daytime sleepiness, inattention, hyperactivity, irritability, and emotional and behavior problems are common.

Unlike the other restless sleep disorders, restless legs syndrome occurs when a person is awake, usually when still and trying to fall asleep or return to sleep. Among children with restless legs syndrome, up to 64 percent have comorbid ADHD, anxiety, depression, and/or behavior problems. This syndrome is not diagnosed by an overnight sleep study, but by self-report (or the report of a parent). It is characterized by four symptoms: Experiencing a weird feeling or strong urge to move the legs, the urge is worse at rest, it's worse in the evening, and it gets better with movement. These strange sensations are difficult for most children and teens to describe, let alone those who are neurodiverse and have communication challenges. In my practice, I've heard this feeling described as many things: a zapping feeling, energy, spiders or bugs crawling around, creepy-crawlies, bees buzzing on the legs, the bones crackling, and feeling like the legs are breaking glass. One research study of kids describing their symptoms included drawings that showed the legs stretching or with zigzags or circles to indicate the unusual feelings. No difference was found in the drawings or descriptions between children with ADHD and those without.[19]

Because restless legs syndrome is unusual and difficult to describe, if we don't ask, kids may not think to tell us about these peculiar feelings. On the other hand, we don't want to ask in a way that encourages a child or teen to say yes. I typically ask, "Is there anything that bothers you when you're trying to fall asleep?" Here I get lots of cute answers, including, "Yes! My feelings because my mommy won't stay in my bed." Then I follow up with, "How about in your body, like arms, legs, or tummy?"

When I think about the complexities of diagnosing RLS, two particular teenagers come to mind: The first was a fifteen-year-old who had just finished years of chemotherapy for bone cancer and was in remission. At bedtime, she would walk around the house continuously. She might get into bed here and there, but she mostly walked around the house again and again until she was so tired she finally passed out wherever she happened to be. Her parents (and I) attributed this to anxiety about her cancer returning and to the trauma of her illness. We thought it was psychological.

The second was an eighteen-year-old neurodiverse young man without a specific diagnosis. He did online college at home, and during or between classes, he would get up and pace around for fifteen to thirty minutes. "I just love pacing!" he told me with a big smile. To calm down at bedtime, he alternated writing pages of numbers with pacing until he, too, finally fell asleep on the couch or his bed.

Though psychological, developmental, and/or medical explanations are possible for these symptoms, it's critical to ask about symptoms of RLS. In each of these cases, after asking more specific questions, I realized that both teenagers had restless legs syndrome.

All three restless sleep disorders relate to low iron stores, measured by a serum ferritin level. If a child or teen has a serum ferritin level below 50 ng/mL, they are treated first with iron supplementation at a dose prescribed by a medical provider. However, most blood testing labs and doctors who aren't sleep specialists consider a serum ferritin level of 50 ng/mL or lower to be normal in terms of "healthy blood." While blood may be healthy, a number of 50 ng/mL or lower is associated with restless sleep, especially in children. The iron supplement is usually oral (liquid or tablet), but if the symptoms cause extreme disruption or if the child cannot tolerate taking iron by mouth, iron can be given intravenously. In fact, with IV iron, symptoms improve immediately, whereas oral iron can take one to three months to work. Further, oral iron tastes bad, stains the teeth, and causes constipation. So why wouldn't everyone get IV iron? To state the obvious, an IV involves a needle stick. Plus, many hospitals and outpatient offices do not yet have protocols for giving IV iron to treat restless sleep disorders.

Circadian Rhythm Sleep Disorders

The internal circadian rhythm of neurodiverse children and teens is often misaligned with the typical twenty-four-hour rhythm, which increases the likelihood of developing a circadian rhythm sleep disorder. Factors contributing to this misalignment include differences in the timing and amount of melatonin secretion, differences in light perception, sensory sensitivities, and other sleep disorders.[20] Circadian rhythm dysfunction also frequently accompanies rare genetic conditions.

Delayed sleep/wake phase disorder occurs when a person's body is ready for sleep much later than typical or ideal for their age. If given the chance, they will also wake up much later. Most of us can't move our own work schedules, nor can we change our child's school, therapy, and activity schedules, to align with their preferred circadian rhythm. But if the child could sleep when their body wanted to sleep, there would be no problem.

For adolescents, there is an additional contributing factor, which is a normal two-hour phase shift that happens near puberty.[21] This delay happens for adolescents all over the world, and for some adolescent animals as well! Teens may not feel sleepy at their previous, earlier bedtime, and they become sleepier during the day. This is a bummer because society hasn't adapted to this delay, so teens not only fall asleep later, but they still must start their school days early. Kudos to districts that have moved middle and high school start times later.

In addition, there is also an advanced sleep/wake phase disorder where people fall asleep much earlier and start their days much earlier than ideal. Imagine falling asleep at 5 p.m. and waking for the day at 2 a.m. This is typically only seen in older adults and in children and adolescents with rare genetic syndromes or medical conditions.

The inconsistent, unpredictable, or erratic circadian rhythm that we sometimes see in neurodiverse kids, especially those with ASD, is called irregular sleep/wake rhythm disorder. For people with this sleep disorder, there is no consistent, internal, established circadian rhythm. They have trouble sleeping for any defined, big chunk of time at night. They are sleepy and often sleep during the day. As the word *irregular* implies, the primary feature is unpredictability.

Occasionally, the circadian clock is free running, moving a little bit every day (called non-24-hour sleep/wake rhythm disorder). This is usually due to visual impairment with an inability to perceive light, but it can also happen in sighted people. One night a person might feel very sleepy at 10 p.m., the next night at 10:30 p.m., then 11 p.m., and so on. The rhythm just keeps following this pattern around the clock.

The American Academy of Sleep Medicine recommends the use of strategically timed melatonin and bright-light therapy (at or above 10,000 lux) in combination with behavioral therapy for children and teens with circadian disorders.[22] Using melatonin and bright-light therapy to shift someone's circadian rhythm should only be done in conjunction with a sleep provider. If the timing isn't correct, the problem can easily get worse and more difficult to treat, so don't go it alone. If you need help finding a sleep specialist, check the resources listed at the end of this chapter; sleep providers are licensed by state, and some see families virtually.

Excessive Daytime Sleepiness

For us sleep nerds, there is a clear distinction between tiredness and sleepiness that doesn't really exist outside of the sleep world. Sleepiness is the propensity to fall asleep. We are sleepy if we could unquestionably take a nap right now. If we feel low energy and would like to lie down but probably wouldn't sleep, then we are tired or fatigued. In general, fatigue is caused by problems other than sleep disorders, such as hypothyroidism, anemia, or depression. Most cases of daytime sleepiness are related to not getting enough sleep or to a sleep disorder that interferes with nighttime sleep quality, such as obstructive sleep apnea or periodic limb movement disorder.

Disorders of excessive daytime sleepiness are uncommon. Two such disorders, narcolepsy and idiopathic hypersomnia, though still very rare, have symptoms that sometimes overlap with neurodevelopmental conditions like ADHD and ASD. Daytime sleepiness, trouble falling asleep, fragmented sleep, and problems with executive functioning are frequent in people with idiopathic hypersomnia and narcolepsy, *and* these symptoms are also common in people with neurodevelopmental conditions. Narcolepsy is thought to be caused by a deficiency in a neurotransmitter called orexin (aka hypocretin), which influences wakefulness. Though we know what narcolepsy looks like and how to treat it, it is difficult to pinpoint a specific cause in most cases. It may be genetic, an autoimmune reaction, or the result of a brain tumor or infection.

Both of these conditions can only be diagnosed with an

overnight sleep study followed by a daytime nap study the next day. Additionally, if a child takes any psychotropic medication (such as for ADHD, anxiety, or depression), it is recommended to consult with a sleep provider well in advance of the sleep study. Often it is recommended to wean certain medications one to six weeks prior to the study, and under the guidance of a physician. This can be a tough choice, especially if those medications are helping a child function. Conducting a study without stopping medications is occasionally done, but idiopathic hypersomnia or narcolepsy might be hidden by either the medication or a rebound immediately after stopping the medication. Discuss the pros and cons with a sleep provider and with the person prescribing any of your child's psychotropic medications.

Idiopathic hypersomnia is a sleep disorder of persistent fatigue and sleepiness. People with idiopathic hypersomnia rarely feel refreshed no matter how long they sleep, even if it's twelve to fourteen hours.

On the other hand, people with narcolepsy might feel great when they wake from a good night of sleep or a nap, but they have the urge to go back to sleep multiple times a day, even in the most exciting situations. Cataplexy, the muscle weakness brought on by strong emotions, is a telltale symptom of narcolepsy (though narcolepsy can occur without cataplexy). Other symptoms of narcolepsy are sleep paralysis and auditory or visual hallucinations when falling asleep (hypnogogic hallucinations) or when waking up (hypnopompic hallucinations). People may see shadowy figures or hear strange noises that aren't really there. Children and teens who experience cataplexy, sleep paralysis, or hallucinations are often scared and confused because they can't control or explain these unusual symptoms. They can't stop their face from drooping, their knees from buckling, or their arm from going limp. They can't physically move from their bed for several minutes, even with a blaring alarm.

A very important caveat is that sleep deprivation also can cause sleep paralysis and/or hypnogogic hallucinations. That is just as scary, but it is not narcolepsy. If your child or teen has any of these unusual symptoms, my advice is for them to be evaluated by a sleep physician. Treatment of both narcolepsy and idiopathic hypersomnia typically includes scheduled naps throughout the day and medications. Medications target either cataplexy or sleepiness, and many people with narcolepsy need both.

While not associated with any specific neurodevelopmental conditions, Kleine-Levin syndrome is another extremely uncommon sleep disorder that occurs most often in white male adolescents or young adults.[23] A person with this syndrome might sleep from fifteen to twenty-one hours in a twenty-four-hour period. This excessive sleep may happen in conjunction with an urgent drive to eat, sexual talk or behavior, cognitive distortions, and apathy, or feeling disconnected from reality. This behavior lasts for several weeks, and after the episode, the person goes right back to sleeping, eating, and behaving exactly the way they did before. People with Kleine-Levin syndrome may have several of these episodes per year, which tend to become shorter, less frequent, and less severe over time before stopping completely.

All three of these rare disorders are usually recognized in adolescence, though symptoms may have been present for much longer. They are frequently misdiagnosed as depression, laziness, substance abuse, and so on. Unfortunately, most people diagnosed with disorders of sleepiness are put through rounds of tests before they make their way to a sleep provider who can untangle their unusual symptoms. One wonderful organization that can help you make sense of these types of rare disorders of excessive sleepiness is Project Sleep (see the resources section at the end of this book).

Next Steps

Medical sleep problems, though rare in the general population, are more common in people with neurodevelopmental conditions.

Parents often ask me if their child's sleep problem is medical or behavioral, and I think what they're really asking is whether they caused their child's sleep problem. It's especially difficult to put sleep symptoms in a single category when working with a neurodivergent child or adolescent, and often it doesn't change the treatment. Behavioral approaches are frequently used to help with medical sleep problems. For example, behavioral techniques are used to help children and teens with obstructive sleep apnea get used to PAP and to help those with delayed sleep/wake phase disorder shift circadian rhythms.

When is the right time to seek professional sleep help, and where do you go? If your child snores, gasps, has pauses in breathing, or complains of a headache upon waking that resolves on its own, an overnight sleep study (PSG; described on page 41) is recommended and can sometimes be ordered by your child's pediatrician. If your child is falling asleep during the day even after getting an appropriate amount of sleep at night, if they complain of weird feelings in their legs, or if they have muscle weakness with emotion, discuss your child's symptoms with their pediatrician, neurologist, or developmental pediatrician.

Many families live in areas without medical specialists nearby. Luckily, many sleep providers have virtual practices. To find a sleep physician, sleep psychologist, sleep nurse practitioner, or physician's assistant licensed in your state, visit one of the following websites to find providers who practice in your region or offer virtual visits:

- American Academy of Sleep Medicine, Sleep Center Directory: https://sleepeducation.org/sleep-center
- Society for Behavioral Sleep Medicine, member directory: https://www.behavioralsleep.org/index.php/united-states -sbsm-members
- Pediatric Sleep Council, Sleep Centers: https://www.baby sleep.com/tools/find-a-sleep-center

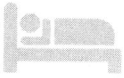

Tuck-In Tips

- Most neurodiverse children and teens are at higher risk of medical sleep disorders.
- If your child snores, they need an overnight sleep study. If possible, have this done at a pediatric sleep lab.
- Strange movements and behaviors during sleep are usually normal, and your child will grow out of them. If you are concerned, video the event and show your pediatrician.
- If your child has episodes of sleepwalking, sleep terrors, or confusional arousals, monitor their safety, increase nighttime sleep, and intervene as little as possible during the event.
- Restless sleep disorders in children can be related to low serum ferritin levels. Consult a sleep provider if you suspect restlessness is interfering with your child's sleep.
- Neurodiverse children and teens often have circadian rhythms misaligned with school schedules, which increases the risk of circadian rhythm sleep disorders.
- Using melatonin and light therapy to shift circadian rhythms should only be done in consultation with a sleep provider, as problems can easily become worse.
- If your child gets enough sleep at night and is old enough not to need a nap, falling asleep during the day is a red flag and should be discussed with your child's pediatrician.

Pillow Point

Symptoms of medical sleep disorders include excessive daytime sleepiness, snoring, restlessness, unusual feelings in the legs, and strange behaviors during sleep. An overnight sleep study (polysomnogram, PSG) is typically required for a diagnosis.

Chapter 6

What If It's Not a
Medical Sleep Disorder?

When I was a postdoctoral fellow in sleep research at the University of Pennsylvania, an incredibly accomplished friend and colleague came to me for help. He and his partner had a toddler with frequent night wakings that were causing the family serious exhaustion, and one of them recently had a fender bender because of it. Their daughter slept in her crib in her room until she started yelling at some point during the night. Then they brought her into their bed, and she went back to sleep until morning. This would not be considered a sleep disorder, or even a problem, unless they did not want her in their bed, and they unequivocally did not. I gave them lots of encouragement and a plan for gradually teaching her to stay in her crib all night. For days, my friend came to work with dark rings around his eyes, and eventually he admitted they couldn't be consistent with the plan. They didn't want a new or different plan, but they just weren't ready. A few weeks later, he pulled me aside to let me know his in-laws were visiting from overseas in two weeks, and if they didn't fix their little one's sleep before that, it would be a disaster for the whole family. So we switched the plan to fast mode.

Faster can also mean more protesting, fussing, and yelling, but even so, for some families, fast is the only way to go. For others, the best plan is to slowly and steadily move the child to their own bed with minimal upset. Still other families plan to co-sleep and have a family bed for years and years. Guess what? *It is all OK.* Though some people feel very strongly one way or the other — that either co-sleeping or not co-sleeping will ruin a child for life — neither of these extremes are well supported by science. I'd love to say that working with a behavioral sleep medicine psychologist yields kind, thoughtful, secure, content, loving, sweet, happy, and generous adults, but darn it, science has not shown that, either. My belief about sleep practices is this: Do what works for everyone in your family to *safely* sleep as well as they can. Then don't feel guilty about the arrangement. Co-sleep safely, don't co-sleep, use white noise or rain sounds, plug in a red nightlight or a blue nightlight: These choices aren't likely to change your child's path in life.

The morning after my friend started the fast sleep plan, he came to me looking more exhausted than ever. The first night had been rough, and although his toddler hadn't been crying much, she did yell for quite a long time, and my friend had doubts.

"Are you sure about this?" he asked. "I mean, this stuff you're telling me, it's just your ideas, right? It's not like it comes from science. This isn't, like, based on research, is it?"

The sleep deprivation was really messing with his brain because what was he thinking? We were in a *sleep research training program*! Someone can be a genius physician who saves lives on the regular and still lose their mind when it comes to their child's sleep. I reassured him that our plan had a solid research foundation comprised of hundreds of scientific studies from as far back as the 1950s, and his determination to stick with the plan was renewed. I was secretly rolling my eyes, but my friend should have been the one rolling *his* eyes at *me*. While I had a good understanding of the research, I had no idea how it feels to teach your own toddler to sleep independently.

Due to our schedules, we didn't see each other for a few weeks.

The next time I saw my friend, he jogged to catch up with me. "Melisa, you'll never believe this!" he said. "We did exactly what you told us to do, and it worked! My daughter falls asleep at 7:30 p.m. and sleeps all night! Can you believe it?"

I laughed that he was so shocked that these techniques worked for his family. Now that I'm a mom, I intimately understand the difference between knowing the science and living it. Regardless, at the time I felt the same way I do now. I felt awesome. There's nothing like helping someone get a good night's sleep.

In the case of my friend's daughter, there wasn't a medical sleep disorder causing her sleep difficulties. Many times there isn't, in which case we look for a behaviorally based sleep disorder. People tend to act embarrassed or ashamed when their kids have a behavioral sleep disorder. I usually hear something like, "I know, I know, it's probably behavioral and my fault." Or, "I've tried everything and I don't see how this could possibly be behavioral." Or, "I'm sorry but we just couldn't take it anymore and we needed sleep." As I mentioned earlier, behavioral sleep problems do not equal terrible parenting. There is no way that the almost 90 percent of neurodiverse kids with sleep issues have bad parents! Nonmedical sleep problems are about associations, habits, and connections in the brain, and the most common example of this in neurodiverse kids is insomnia.

Insomnia

Insomnia involves difficulty falling asleep, difficulty staying asleep, and/or waking too early. And if we put together all the studies of insomnia in people along the whole spectrum of neurodivergence, it's clear that nearly everyone has it. To diagnose insomnia disorder, a child or their parent must report that the symptoms are problematic. I might see a family where the parents happily sing and rock their child for thirty minutes with a bottle until they fall asleep. The child may wake throughout the night and need the parent to provide a few sips of the bottle, and everyone is OK with it. This is a sleep association, but it's not insomnia disorder. If I see another family with the same routine, and they are begging me to help with their child's night wakings because everyone is exhausted, that is insomnia.

Insomnia develops from a combination of internal and external factors, which are referred to as the three P's: predisposing, precipitating, and perpetuating. The "3P" model has been around forever (or at least since 1986) and is still standing, and it's been studied in adults, children, and teens.[1]

As for the three P's, *predisposing* factors are generally internal factors, or things we are born with, like neurodiversity! Another big one is preference for night versus day. Your child or teen might naturally be a night owl, or they might be an early bird. Regardless, this circadian preference must be managed so the child can go to school, be with friends, and participate in activities. *Precipitating* factors are events that trigger the sleep problem, like moving, welcoming a new sibling, an upcoming doctor's appointment or test, an argument with a friend, or some cause we have no idea about. Henry has insomnia whenever he gets a new toy, plays a new game, or has a new idea. I remember having a very cool car shaped like a tiger in my pocket to reward Henry for getting through a dreaded haircut. I knew it would make the haircut a million times easier, but I also knew the risk of sleep disruption that would follow. Haircut or sleep is one tough choice. *Perpetuating* factors are things that keep the insomnia going, such as a sleep association that involves another person, adding an extra nap to compensate for difficulty falling asleep, or making bedtime earlier. For a summary, see table 6.1.

Table 6.1: The Three P's That Contribute to Insomnia

Predisposing Factors that make insomnia more likely	Precipitating Events that trigger insomnia	Perpetuating Factors that keep insomnia going
• Genetics • Early infancy (still developing circadian system) • Adolescence (circadian delay) • ADHD • ASD • Anxiety • Depression • Pain • Night/day preference • Medical issues • Personality traits	• Developmental milestones • School stress • Change or transition • Illness or medical condition • Medication • Living situation • Neighborhood noise • School, work, or therapy schedule • Sensory sensitivities • Stimming	• Sleep association • Parental presence at bedtime • Earlier bedtime • Weekend oversleep • Napping • Caffeine

Many times, even when predisposing factors like anxiety or pain improve, insomnia lingers and needs to be specifically and directly addressed. Cognitive behavioral therapy for insomnia is the current gold standard of treatment. This is short-term therapy (typically two to twelve sessions) focused on improving sleep habits, managing unhelpful thoughts and beliefs about sleep, increasing sleep pressure, and retraining the brain that the bed is only for sleep. Since I primarily work with children, my approach is generally lighter on the cognitive and heavier on the behavioral. It's impossible for a two-year-old to reflect on their own unhelpful thoughts about sleep. Their brain can't do that yet! I use this therapy as the foundation for most of what I do because it has strong scientific support in a variety of people with a range of conditions and in different environments. My approach looks different for different families, but it all starts at the same place.

CHANGES IN ROUTINE

If your child is sick or scared, you have visitors, you take a trip, or if anything else temporarily disrupts your child's sleep, don't worry about briefly changing the routine. Even babies learn that there are different rules for different situations. Once your circumstances return to normal, go right back to your typical home bedtime rules ASAP. The first few nights may be challenging, but sleep should get better in a few days by communicating the expectations and consistently following the steps of the regular routine.

Nighttime Fears

Nighttime fears are technically neither sleep disorders nor anxiety disorders, but they relate to both. Children with neurodevelopmental conditions are more likely to have comorbid anxiety, and sometimes that anxiety sparks nighttime fears. Neurodiverse kids and teens sometimes have difficulty understanding expectations around sleep, and this also can cause nighttime fears (see chapter 10). Finally, a child may be used to sleeping with a parent, and when the parent goes back to their own bed, the child is afraid to be alone. While parental presence generally alleviates nighttime fears temporarily, after several nights, an unwanted sleep association can develop.

The hard part about nighttime fears is that the way to move past them is to face them, which is not at all appealing to a scared child. Facing fears means teaching our brain that we will not be eaten by a monster during the night...by repeatedly experiencing a monster not eating us at night. In chapter 15, I share some tips and tricks to help your child gradually face nighttime fears.

Tuck-In Tips

- Almost all neurodiverse people experience insomnia (trouble falling asleep, staying asleep, or waking too early).
- For a diagnosis of insomnia disorder, the child and/or parent must report that the symptoms bother them.
- Insomnia results from predisposing, precipitating, and perpetuating factors (the three P's).
- Nighttime fears interfere with sleep and can be related to anxiety. Gradually facing fears helps to alleviate them.

Pillow Point

Almost all neurodivergent children, teens, and adults experience insomnia.

Chapter 7

What If the Sleep Problem Isn't Caused by a Sleep Disorder?

A mom I was working with once emailed me, "Just changed a poopy diaper that Levi insisted he had, which he didn't, and I even pretended to clean up poop from his crib that he said was there, which it wasn't. All in the name of trying to get him back to sleep. It's so annoying and so funny at the same time and hard to set limits when potty training....He really is convinced it is a poop and even makes me wipe it off the mattress! What should I do?"

In addition to sleep, toileting is often challenging for neurodiverse kids, and it's hard to know what to prioritize! Prolonged ignoring isn't a good solution in the case of poop. The day you pretend it's not happening is the day you walk into your child's room after naptime to find the walls finger painted brown or your child's bum with a painful diaper rash that lasts for days and causes even more problems for sleep.

I am lucky because both my kids have almost always pooped at the same time, right before bedtime, ever since they've been potty trained. This just happened; it wasn't something I planned. Kids are trained to hold it, but training a person to *go* is a different story. Our poop timing evolved because of our bedtime routine. Snack was (and still is) first, then sit on the toilet, have a bath or shower, brush teeth, and so on. Since they were babies, my kids have loved mangos, strawberries, pears, or pretty much any fruit, and they often choose this for bedtime snack. In the past, if bedtime was running behind, the kids might just slurp back an apple juice box. Fruit and apple juice both tend to move things along, and so our kids usually had some toileting success within ten minutes of sitting down. I'm grateful for this every time I work with kids whose painful constipation gets in the way of a good night's sleep. Occasionally, parents get a break, and things like poop schedules go the right way without doing anything!

Medical Sleep Thieves

While not a sleep disorder, constipation is just one medical condition that causes sleep problems. There are many medical and psychological conditions that aren't in themselves sleep disorders, yet they get in the way of sleep. The most common medical sleep thieves in neurodiverse kids are gastrointestinal problems, allergies, asthma, eczema, and seizures. The belly can be the biggest headache when it comes to sleep, and about 75 percent of kids with ADHD, ASD, and Down syndrome have gastrointestinal troubles.

Of these, the most common problems for neurodiverse kids are gastroesophageal reflux disease (GERD), constipation, and irritable bowel syndrome. GERD is when stomach acid repeatedly flows back up through the esophagus and causes heartburn, pain, coughing, and/or a backwash of food and sour liquid in the throat and mouth. GERD is worse lying down, it can be very painful and disruptive to sleep, and it tends to be most apparent in the first few hours of sleep. While eating and drinking may initially be soothing, GERD can cause spit up or vomiting, which eventually can lead to an empty stomach and hunger, causing the cycle to start again with eating. Things that improve GERD include sitting upright for thirty minutes after eating, medications, avoiding certain foods, and timing of eating relative to lying down. A bedtime snack right before lying down is *not* a recommended part of the bedtime routine for children and teens with GERD.

Constipation and irritable bowel syndrome are common in more than half of neurodiverse kids, especially those who are selective eaters. Both conditions can be especially uncomfortable at night. Constipation is not only a big pain, but it can also cause big pain, while irritable bowel syndrome can involve diarrhea, constipation, or alternating between both. Treatments include medications, exercise, dietary changes, and scheduled sitting on the toilet.

Our gut biome is the ecosystem within our gastrointestinal system made up of bacteria, viruses, parasites, fungi, and other teeny tiny microorganisms, and there is a connection between this gut biome and neurodevelopmental conditions such as ADHD, ASD, and Down syndrome. However, in my opinion, there isn't enough research to be able to say exactly *how* they relate to each other.[1] Definitely don't believe what you read on the internet, where claims abound that a child's neurodiversity might have been caused by the mother having a C-section, or the use of antibiotics, or not giving an infant probiotics, or feeding a baby formula, and so on. Science does not support those claims.

Separately, eczema, asthma, and allergies are interconnected medical issues that are related to each other, to neurodiversity, and to sleep.[2] Someone with asthma or allergies is more likely to have eczema, someone with eczema or asthma is more likely to have allergies,[3] and someone with any of these is more likely to be neurodivergent and to have sleep problems. Even if the itching, coughing, snoring, or disrupted breathing doesn't seem to wake your child or teen enough for you to hear about it, it is still waking their developing brain and diminishing their sleep quality.

There are also complex relationships among seizures, sleep, and neurodiversity. Children with ADHD, ASD, Angelman syndrome, and some other neurodevelopmental conditions have higher rates of epilepsy. Not only do seizures cause disrupted sleep, but disrupted or insufficient sleep can cause seizures. It's a serious situation that can interfere with the entire family's sleep. When a child or teen has seizures, often the parents sleep during the day or in shifts, so they can watch their child for signs of a seizure at night, at least until the seizures are controlled with medications. There is an incredible amount of pressure on parents of children with epilepsy to make sure their children get the best possible sleep to avoid provoking a seizure. I want to acknowledge how stressful that can be. My best advice is to strategize how everyone can get the best sleep most often. That might mean asking friends or family for help, taking turns with a partner, or using a baby monitor — and buy a new one if your child is older, since the technology has really advanced.

On top of those medical problems, medications can cause trouble falling asleep *or* they can cause sleepiness. For example, the oral steroids used to treat an asthma flare can cause hyperactivity and muck up sleep. Taking stimulant medications too late in the day can lead to extra energy and problems falling asleep (though sometimes they can help sleep). When comparing children with ADHD on stimulants versus those off stimulants, no significant sleep differences have been found.[4] In other words, stimulant medications don't inherently make sleep better or worse, but the timing can be a factor. On the other hand, taking sedating medications such as antihistamines during the day can lead to excessive daytime napping, which then takes away sleep pressure and makes it harder to fall asleep at night. For most medicines that cause sleep problems, the way to make sleep better is to discontinue them. However, don't immediately stop a child's medications without talking to their medical provider. Some medications need to be tapered slowly before stopping.

Neurodiverse kids are complicated, and parents try to make all the systems in their life the best they can be. But it's too much to attempt everything simultaneously: potty training, sleep training, increasing the span of preferred foods, and learning to put on shoes, zip up a coat, swallow pills, say a new word, and so on. It's impossible for your child (and for you) to work on everything at once. Use your child's team to help you prioritize. For me, after safety and acute medical concerns, sleep is usually the top priority. Of course, at times I focus less on sleep and more on school or mood or nutrition or finding a special-needs baseball team. Most often, though, sleep is at the top of my list because I love sleep, and everyone in my house, including me, needs it to function.

Psychological Sleep Thieves

Up to 85 percent of neurodiverse kids have comorbid psychological diagnoses, and this is a double whammy for sleep. In children and adolescents with ADHD and/or ASD, the rates of all psychological conditions are higher, from obsessive-compulsive disorder to depression to conduct disorder to tics. Neurodiverse kids with psychological comorbidities also have higher rates of sleep problems.

Psychological conditions can be divided into internalizing and externalizing disorders. Internalizing disorders occur when the symptoms (withdrawal, sad mood, worries) are directed inward. In neurodiverse kids, mood disorders are the most common psychological diagnoses, and anxiety is the worst offender. Up to 70 percent of youth with ASD have clinically significant anxiety, and up to 64 percent of children with ADHD have at least one diagnosed anxiety disorder.[5] These include generalized anxiety disorder (where worries encompass a variety of everyday things), specific phobias, post-traumatic stress disorder, separation anxiety disorder, obsessive-compulsive disorder, and Tourette syndrome. These rates are much higher than the 5 to 15 percent of children and adolescents in the general population who have anxiety disorders. Most anxiety disorders have a two-way relationship with sleep: Anxiety leads to more sleep problems, and sleep problems lead to more anxiety.[6]

Neurodiverse children and teens are also at increased risk for depression.[7] In addition to emotion regulation difficulties, sensory sensitivities, genetic factors, and comorbidities, it is beyond demanding to be neurodivergent in a world designed for neurotypical people. Neurodiverse kids can be irritable and sad, thus decreasing their enjoyment of activities, and they can rely heavily on predictability: They may prefer to eat the same foods, watch the same shows, read the same books, and do the same activities. Neurodiverse kids may return to what they liked to watch, do, or play even several years ago, at times when they need comfort.

Mood disorders (anxiety and depression) in neurodiverse children and teens are underrecognized, underdiagnosed, and undertreated. Figuring out what's what is complicated due to speech and language delays, differences in how the symptoms of anxiety show up, the tendency for providers to focus on whatever the neurodiverse condition is, and/or difficulties neurodiverse kids have verbally communicating emotions.

Many providers view anxiety as a normal part of ASD, and while they often co-occur, they are two distinct conditions. Cognitive behavioral therapy with or without medication is the treatment of choice for mood disorders in children and teens with or without ADHD or ASD.[8] Cognitive behavioral therapy for mood disorders is a focused, time-limited therapy (usually six to twenty sessions). Like cognitive behavioral therapy for insomnia, the focus is on identifying unhelpful thoughts, beliefs, and behaviors to improve mood. Traditional techniques may need to be adapted for neurodivergent kids and teens, so if possible, seek out a therapist who has experience treating mood disorders in the context of neurodiversity.

Externalizing disorders include oppositional defiant disorder, conduct disorder, and disruptive behavior disorders. ADHD itself is considered an externalizing disorder, though in this book I'm approaching it as a neurodevelopmental condition. These are categorized as "externalizing" because the symptoms (testing limits, impulsivity, hyperactivity, aggression) are directed outward or externally. We can usually see and hear these behaviors loud and clear. Up to 70 percent of children diagnosed with ASD also have ADHD, and while they are considered distinct disorders, there is high symptom overlap.[9] Similarly, children and teens diagnosed with oppositional defiant disorder compared with those diagnosed with ASD show similar behaviors (tantrums, defiance), but for different reasons. One child may be challenging authority while the other may be reacting to sensory overload. Externalizing disorders also have a two-way relationship with sleep.[10] For example, oppositional defiant disorder might increase the risk of bedtime resistance and bedtime tantrums, causing a late bedtime and insufficient sleep. Insufficient sleep might lead to increased irritability and disruptive behaviors.

A major underlying cause of comorbid psychological disorders in neurodiverse kids is emotional dysregulation. Studies have shown that neurodiverse or not, poor sleep leads to impairments in the processing of emotions. Sleep-deprived children and adolescents express less emotion overall, express more negative emotions, use fewer positive emotion words, and show more negative facial expressions. Children and teens who don't sleep well show less prosocial behavior, less satisfaction with friendships, and more negative peer interactions. The effect is even greater if they have preexisting anxiety. Neurodiverse kids may already have difficulties with emotion regulation and social skills. Geez, can neurodiverse kids catch a break?

Irritability is another factor that relates to both psychological problems and sleep problems.[11] Irritability is "in-the-moment" anger, grouchiness, prickliness, crabbiness, or grumpiness that is not proportionate to the situation. Children and teens who are neurodiverse are more likely to be irritable; their reactions are often bigger than the situation calls for. Neurodiverse kids have a lot to be irritable about: sensory sensitivities, difficulty with transitions, a day full of nonpreferred activities, executive-function challenges, social challenges, unpredictability, you name it. Then there's sleep. Not getting enough sleep, poor-quality sleep, trouble sleeping, and daytime sleepiness are irritating! This is worst in the morning when waking from a rough night of sleep. There is scientific evidence that the relationship between sleep and irritability is both important and distinct in neurodiverse kids. It's not just that poor sleep leads to poor emotional regulation, which leads to irritability. Poor sleep also directly causes irritability, and irritability directly causes poor sleep. When was the last time you were irritable and had an easy time falling asleep?

Whew! There are a lot of medical and psychological problems that are common in neurodiverse kids *and cause sleep problems.* So many. Fixing those is a priority, but you don't have to wait for constipation to fully resolve or for a spider phobia to be all gone before working on sleep. In some cases, when the non-sleep problem is fixed, the sleep gets better; however, often the sleep problem persists and needs direct treatment. This goes back to sleep associations. Think about pain. When pain gets in the way of sleep for several nights, an association between lying down and pain begins to override the more helpful association between lying down and sleep. Eventually, lying down signals the brain that pain, not sleep, is on its way, and the brain becomes primed for pain. Chapters 13 and 14 address changing sleep associations.

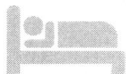

Tuck-In Tips

- Many medical conditions get in the way of good sleep for neurodiverse kids. The most common are gastrointestinal problems, allergies, asthma, eczema, and seizures.
- Neurodiverse people have higher rates of almost all psychological comorbidities, from anxiety to disruptive behavior disorders, and this is partially explained by difficulty regulating emotions.

- For neurodiverse kids, irritability is a key symptom of mood disorders and/or poor sleep.
- Treating the underlying medical or psychological problem is a priority, but it may not fix the sleep problem. Often the sleep problem needs to be treated separately.

Pillow Point

The medical and psychological problems common in neurodiverse kids also cause sleep problems, yet even when the underlying problem is resolved, sleep often has to be treated directly.

Chapter 8

Does This Stuff Apply to Children with Rare Conditions?

Sleep problems in rare diagnoses are not only a result of the condition, but they are also caused by the jumble of medical and behavioral sleep disorders described in chapters 5 and 6. The family of Willa, a seventeen-year-old girl with a yet-unnamed genetic syndrome, came to our sleep clinic because she could not fall asleep or return to sleep without her mom. If Mom tried to leave while Willa was awake, even for a quick trip to the bathroom, Willa would bang her head on the wall or pull out her hair. Medications had been suggested by Willa's developmental pediatrician; however, that received an instant no from her parents. She'd had an adverse reaction to a sleep medication years ago wherein she was awake and agitated for a dreadful forty-eight hours, and her parents did not want to relive it. They asked me for behavioral recommendations.

Willa's sleep problems had been going on for years, so why did the family seek help now? I find out so much important information by asking that question. Willa had been fed by g-tube (or feeding tube) for several years, and during that time, home nursing was present about five nights per week. Having a nurse at night allowed Willa's parents to sleep for seven to eight hours four to five times per week because they didn't have to monitor her g-tube. When I saw the family, Willa was eating so well by mouth that her g-tube had been removed. While this was fantastic, it also meant that Willa's family lost night nursing as well as their own consistent sleep.

Two to four times each night, Willa cried and patted her diaper to show it was wet. Mom came in, turned on a dim lamp, and changed the diaper, though it was almost always dry. She gave Willa extra snuggles, another tuck in, and a sip of water. If the diaper did need to be changed, it was usually a poop, the room was stinky, and Mom turned on a lavender diffuser to cover the smell. The times Mom didn't go into Willa's room right away, Willa began banging her head and pulling her hair again. Willa had a helmet prescribed by her neurologist for similar daytime behaviors. Her parents occasionally put it on her at night until she calmed down and stopped hurting herself, but she did not sleep with it. The helmet not only prevented a head injury, but it was comforting to Willa. These were rough times for the family, and Willa's mom in particular was sleep-deprived, depressed, and frequently sick.

The sleep center staff recognized this family's desperation and the whole team rallied. One of our nurses spoke with the home nursing and the insurance companies to see if night nursing could be restarted, and they said no. I reached out to Willa's neurologist to see if she could wear the helmet all night. He said no because it was a safety risk. We were stuck. One of the sleep physicians (also a psychiatrist) talked to Willa's parents about starting an antidepressant, sertraline, which can also reduce anxiety. Willa's parents asked all their questions about the medication, and they developed a plan in case Willa had another unpredictable reaction. They felt comfortable with Willa trying a low dose, and they agreed to consider giving Willa melatonin in the future. The psychology team also helped Willa's mom find a psychiatrist for herself.

Three months later, Willa and her parents returned to the sleep clinic. The sertraline was working miracles. Willa was no longer injuring herself during the day, she seemed happier, and she was making incredible progress communicating. Unfortunately, her sleep had not improved, and it became clear that Willa's crying about her dry diaper was being reinforced by Mom's positive attention. Together, we decided that, after Willa's mom went to sleep at 10 p.m., Willa's dad would take over sleep duty. He would check Willa's diaper when she cried, but he'd do this quickly, with no talking and no additional light, tuck in, snuggles, or lavender diffuser. Afterward, he held up the water bottle to offer a sip, and then he sat silently in the room until Willa returned to sleep. If she started hurting herself, he put on her helmet. When she was calm, he took off the helmet and gave her a favorite stuffed rabbit.

I saw the family about two months later, and Willa's sleep was finally getting better. A few weeks after I had last seen them, Willa's mom got Covid and was too sick to get out of bed for four nights. Dad was unable to sit in Willa's room at bedtime or during the night due to needing to work and sleep. In an effort to maximize everyone's sleep on those nights, he gave her a small dose of melatonin at bedtime, and this was immensely helpful. Willa fell asleep more quickly and without a parent sitting in her room. Even after Willa's mom recovered, Willa no longer called for her during the night, which surprised her parents. She still woke for one to two hours each night, but her parents could see on the monitor that she was safe, and eventually she returned to sleep on her own. They wanted to know if the improvement was the result of Willa learning to soothe herself back to sleep or due to the melatonin. My guess is that it was probably both. Willa's bedtime problems and night wakings were likely due to a combination of neurodivergence and negative sleep associations.

Rare Conditions Are Rarely the Only Cause

When I worked at a big urban children's hospital, I sometimes saw "the only one" of something: the only child with a specific genetic deletion, the one-in-a-million disease, the bizarre injury, the extraordinary brain tumor, or the illness most physicians have only seen in a textbook. As a pediatric sleep psychologist, I saw children and teens with the rarest of conditions because sleep relates to everything and everyone. Also, sleep is usually easy to talk about, which is especially welcome in a hospital where difficult conversations are happening around every corner. One of my psychology professors said he always opened the first therapy session with "How's your sleep?" While people are hesitant to share private thoughts and feelings with a stranger, they are rarely defensive about their sleep.

Sleep might relate to everything, but few medical and psychological providers know much about it, and it's not their fault. Psychology and medical trainees (outside of sleep programs) typically have very little education, training, or experience with sleep disorders. Also, medical providers who work in children's hospitals are typically in the business of figuring out what's wrong and making it better. They want to make that diagnosis and recommend a therapy, do a surgery, or prescribe a medication that will fix it. As you might guess, this is not always straightforward when it comes to pediatric sleep problems in the context of neurodevelopmental conditions. I feel incredibly fortunate to have worked alongside some of the smartest, most dedicated, and most genuinely well-intentioned people I've ever met — all my hospital colleagues, both past and present.

And still. Unless they've gone through it, they might not always get it.

I once asked a supervisor how I should respond to parents who ask how I could possibly help them when I hadn't gone through what they were going through. "Does an oncologist have to have cancer to treat cancer?" she asked. "Should your therapist have a history of depression?" Well, no, but as I eventually learned, there is undoubtedly something different about having been there.

When it comes to rare conditions, I've been told by families that it's often hard to feel like you and your child are being seen. I kept that in mind as I planned and wrote this book, since I want it to speak to and help the parent of *any* neurodiverse child with sleep problems. As such, I wanted to include every condition, common or rare, with published research associated with both sleep problems and neurodiversity in children. Investigating this led me to identify around fifty rare conditions, which I promptly put into a spreadsheet so that I could compare them in terms of sleep symptoms.

In addition to ADHD, ASD, and Down syndrome, sleep problems are associated with the following rare syndromes, diseases, and disorders: Angelman syndrome, Batten disease, Beckwith-Weidemann syndrome, cerebral palsy, Charcot-Marie-Tooth disease, CHARGE syndrome, Chiari malformations, Cornelia de Lange syndrome, Cri du chat syndrome, Crouzon syndrome, DiGeorge syndrome, fetal alcohol spectrum disorders, Fragile X syndrome, Jacobsen syndrome, Moebius syndrome, mucopolysaccharidosis, muscular dystrophy, neurofibromatosis, Pallister-Killian syndrome, Phelan-McDermid syndrome, Pierre Robin sequence, Prader-Willi syndrome, Rett syndrome, ROHHAD syndrome, Smith-Kingsmore syndrome, Smith-Lemli-Opitz syndrome, Smith-Magenis syndrome, Sotos syndrome, spinal muscular atrophy, Treacher Collins syndrome, tuberous sclerosis, Williams syndrome, and more conditions that I haven't named or that don't yet have names.[1]

Acquired neurodiversities are also very rare. These are the result of an illness, accident, exposure, or other outside event like a birth injury, stroke, brain tumor, traumatic brain injury, toxin exposure, or infection that occurs during or after birth. As a result of the event, physical changes to the brain and brain chemistry alter perception, processing, and expression, causing a new, permanent condition like ADHD or cerebral palsy, which consequently impacts sleep.

Looking at my spreadsheet trying to make sense of the data, I was surprised by what I found. It also made this chapter much shorter than I expected. Whether genetic or acquired, whether similar or radically different from one another, rare conditions tend to be associated with the same sleep disorders: obstructive sleep apnea, circadian rhythm disorders, periodic limb movement disorder, and the biggest one, insomnia disorder.

Taking Action and Getting Help

Sleep problems in neurodivergent kids are complex — and all the more so with rare conditions. So what do you do when you and your child are exhausted from the very sleep problems you need to fix?

Start by doing two things at the same time. First, work with your child's pediatrician or specialist to have a complete evaluation to rule out any comorbid medical or psychological conditions that might also be impacting sleep (like those in chapters 5, 6, and 7). Next, and perhaps more importantly, work on improving your child's overall sleep habits as much as you can (which is the focus of part 2).

This doesn't mean that bad sleep habits are causing the problem or that good sleep hygiene and a consistent schedule will fix the problem, but it's *the* place to start. Not only might it help directly, but it will also guide the providers who are trying to determine the best approach to improving your child's sleep. Make sure to accurately describe what your child's sleep habits are and what you have tried so far. Take pictures of the pages from this book that speak to you and bring them to your child's next appointment. You don't have to follow through with any treatment you don't agree with, but it can be reassuring to know there is almost always something else to try. Here are further specific steps to take:

1. Contact the specialist who diagnosed, treated, or is currently treating your child. Ask about the sleep problems associated with your child's diagnosis. Ask about medications

your child is taking to see if any are known to interfere with sleep.

2. Reach out to experts on your child's diagnosis at other hospitals. In my experience, emailing a nurse, social worker, or administrative assistant on the expert's team often results in an interaction with that expert. Post-Covid, many physicians and psychologists do virtual consults, so even if you aren't in the same geographic area, it's worth making contact.

3. Find societies and associations for your child's condition and join online groups. You can always be anonymous if you aren't ready to share your name. Ask others who have children with the same sleep problem as yours what they have tried.

4. Ask your child's pediatrician, primary care doctor, specialist, or sleep physician if an overnight sleep study (PSG) is indicated for your child's sleep problem. This is the only way obstructive and/or central apnea, periodic limb movement disorder, and restless sleep disorder can be detected. If daytime sleepiness is a problem, your child may also need a daytime nap study, which can often only be ordered by a sleep physician.

5. If your child is restless during sleep, when trying to fall asleep, or when returning to sleep, ask their pediatrician, primary care doctor, or sleep physician about checking a serum ferritin level. Many providers don't know about the association between ferritin and restless sleep, so perhaps take a picture of the information about it in this book (including related sources), or find an article from a reputable source for backup.

6. At some point, consider your child's circadian rhythm. If they are falling asleep and waking up too late, expose them to as much natural sunlight in the morning as you can, make sure they have a consistent wake time, and avoid

all daytime napping. If their circadian rhythm is too early (falling asleep early and waking for the day early), expose your child to natural sunlight later in the afternoon. In all cases, restrict sunlight and avoid electronics from the time they first fall asleep until an acceptable (to you) wake time.

7. Try to feed your child (even if they are fed by tube) at your family's typical breakfast, lunch, and dinner times to cue the circadian cells in the gastrointestinal system.

8. For circadian rhythm problems and insomnia, discuss with your doctor whether melatonin might be an appropriate supplement.

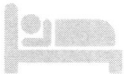

Tuck-In Tips

- Most genetic syndromes and acquired neurodiversities are associated with higher risks of obstructive sleep apnea, periodic limb movement disorder, restless sleep disorder, circadian rhythm disorders, and insomnia.

- Ask your child's pediatrician to evaluate for any medical or psychological conditions that interfere with sleep.

- As best you can, spiff up your child's sleep habits and maintain a consistent schedule and nightly bedtime routine. Let providers know what you have tried.

- Talk to medical, psychological, and parent experts in your child's condition about their experience with sleep problems, and find out what has helped other families.

- Ask your child's pediatrician, specialist, or sleep physician if an overnight sleep study and/or serum ferritin level are indicated.

- Discuss adjusting medications and feedings to align with a typical circadian rhythm.

Pillow Point

Seek out medical, psychological, and parent experts in your child's condition to find out about common sleep issues, and ask a medical provider if an overnight sleep study and/or serum ferritin level would help them to further evaluate your child's sleep.

PART 2

Improving Sleep in Neurodiverse Kids

Chapter 9

Where Should I Start?

I've had more than one exhausted family member ask me if it's possible to die from sleep deprivation. We get through periods of horrible sleep not because the universe only gives people the challenges they are strong enough to handle, and all that other well-meaning blabbity blah. We do it because we have to.

I will never forget one mom who had a daughter with Down syndrome and frequent night wakings. She legitimately wondered if she was facing certain death from being woken every hour from 11 p.m. to 5 a.m. every night. Her three-year-old daughter Mia would only fall asleep and return to sleep while being rocked in a hammock. This started because two years earlier, prior to the hammock, Mia could only sleep being rocked in her mom's tired arms. Since Mia's birth, this supermom had not had a single stretch of sleep longer than two hours, and she was desperate. A family member visiting from Asia brought a free-standing baby hammock, and when Mia was in it, she seemed to sleep better. She still woke every forty-five to ninety minutes, but now Mia's mom could sleep beside her and just reach up and rock the hammock when she woke. This had been the situation for about two years.

I wanted to climb over that hypothetical professional wall, hug her, and say, "I totally get it, sister. You're looking at me and wondering how it is possible to muster the energy to do yet one more thing when you're already sleep-deprived. I'm looking at you wondering how we can get rid of that hammock." Why was that my goal? The problem was that the rocking and the hammock were needed for Mia to calm down and fall asleep. Without them, she couldn't get back to sleep easily on her own during the normal wakings that happen at the end of each sleep cycle.

The other concern I had was safety. Granted, Mia was not a newborn at high risk for sudden infant death syndrome, but she did have low muscle tone. I was worried that the cozy scrunched-up-ness of the hammock might make it harder for her to breathe during sleep. Plus, children with Down syndrome are already at high risk for obstructive sleep apnea. So Mia's mom gradually reduced the rocking, but Mia still couldn't seem to sleep anywhere but that hammock. Then the mom came up with the winning idea: If she hid the baby hammock, her daughter wouldn't be reminded of it. Mia wouldn't be motivated to stay awake until she was rocked to sweet slumber in that hammock if she didn't see it. Could it really be as easy as out of sight, out of mind? I was skeptical that this would be the true end of it, but it was! At this point, Mia was three, and yes, it took her longer to fall asleep in her crib at first. Mom had to pat her back for about two weeks before gradually fading the patting, but hiding the hammock was the key for Mia.

Parents of neurodiverse kids are so smart! Of course, it's hard to be smart when we're too sleep-deprived to think, but this is the place to start: Identify the main problem, your goals, and what might motivate your family to make a change.

Name the Real Problem

First, determine what the bare-bones problem is. I don't mean just for your neurodiverse child; I mean for your whole family, including you. Is the problem that your child is not sleeping ten hours per night, or is the problem that you are not sleeping because you are worried that they might not be safe if they are awake alone? Is the problem that your child is awake for two hours in the middle of the night, or is it that your other children can't sleep because your neurodiverse child is vocalizing loudly for two hours? If, despite wakefulness at night, your child is not falling asleep during the day at school or in their therapies, then the problem might not be your neurodiverse child's sleep. It might be that their particular sleep pattern is normal for them but not for your family. This doesn't mean there isn't a problem. *There is.* It just means that the problem might not be a behavioral or medical *sleep* disorder.

Set a Realistic Goal

After identifying the specific problem, ask yourself what you want to change about the situation, and make that your goal. Personally, it sometimes bugs me when people suggest setting goals, like at the gym. They rarely seem attainable to me. Yeah, I'd love to go to the gym six days a week, but it's just not gonna happen. I'll be lucky if I make it once or twice. How's that for a goal?

As a therapist who has worked with thousands of families, I know goals are important. But make them realistic. Start small with a goal you can reach. Don't base your goals on someone else's idea of what you should do or what your child's sleep should be, unless that person is a pediatric sleep expert or an expert in neurodiverse children like yours. If a preschooler with ASD sleeps for only eight hours at night, but they wake happy and don't sleep during daytime activities, this might be what it is. Often, we have to shift our goals to be aligned with who our neurodiverse child is and what they need. This is where the ideal meets the real.

Here's an example: After Henry started on medications that took away his appetite during the day, he would wake up at night starving, and he'd yell about being hungry until I got him one snack after another. I couldn't bring two snacks at the same time. If I did, he would wake me up repeatedly until I took the second one away because what if he was full from the first one and didn't need the second one? Later, if he was still hungry, he'd call me again for a second or third snack. People generally cannot sleep through hunger, so ignoring Henry wasn't an option. I also knew this wasn't a sustainable pattern for me, and I had to get down to the real issues:

- My child needed a stimulant to function in school, and when he took it, he wasn't hungry during the day.
- When the medication wore off in the evening, he was hungry, and he was also hungry during the night.
- His weight was low.
- He was a picky eater.
- It wasn't healthy for our family to be woken multiple times during the night.

What was the problem? Henry got hungry during the night, and I didn't want to be woken multiple times to get him sequential snacks. What was the goal? For everyone in the family, including me, to get as much sleep as possible. Actual hunger can disrupt sleep. Since I couldn't stop Henry from being hungry, I chose to give him food, but I also set a limit. At bedtime, I left multiple snacks on his bedside dresser, even if he only wanted one at a time. He could eat as little or as much as he wanted, but he had to feed himself, not ask me to bring him food in the middle of the night. It took a week for him to get used to not having Mom-provided sequential snacks. Now during the night when he is motivated by hunger, he independently eats his snacks and (mostly) goes back to sleep on his own.

Of course, he still wakes me up on occasion, such as when he desperately needs to tell me that from now on he only wants watermelon, not grapes, or he needs to ask a burning question, such as, "If a person can't see or hear, what language do they think in?" I know my solution is not in the handbook of perfect parenting. As I describe earlier, Henry should probably brush his teeth after each snack, which should be protein-rich to keep him full longer.

Plus, leaving food in his room might attract insects and pests. But did I achieve my goals? Yes. Maybe our family doesn't get ten uninterrupted hours of sleep every single night, but it is certainly "as much sleep as possible" for right now.

That earns a gold star.

Motivate Your Child with Rewards

If your child is beyond infancy, as you strategize how to improve sleep issues, it's important to ask: What might motivate your neurodiverse child to change? You might wonder if getting better sleep in itself is enough of a reward for your child. Um, no. Children rarely are the ones asking to make an appointment with a pediatric sleep specialist.

While praise and positive responses, such as smiling and clapping, are wonderful ways to provide reinforcement, often parents need to provide additional external motivation, a reward the child truly wants. Sleep motivators or rewards are notoriously tricky. In general, when rewards are used to encourage behavior change, they work best when given ASAP, immediately after the child does what was asked. But lights out is not an ideal time for a fun activity or treat, since that interrupts the process of going to sleep, and rewards for bedtime routines don't always work if given the next morning. Especially for younger children, too much time has passed, and they won't associate the reward with the behavior.

Candy and chocolate are often powerful, easy rewards to give; some kids will do anything for a sweet treat. But it's reasonable to think twice about rewarding your child with chocolate after teeth brushing. You do have to face the dentist, after all. Another consideration is what will happen if your child doesn't earn the promised reward. Will your child become so upset that a long meltdown will ensue, delaying bedtime for hours? It's a challenge to find something that is motivating enough, can be given at bedtime without negative consequences, and won't cause a meltdown if not earned. And oh, by the way, won't make you feel like a terrible parent.

One more tricky thing about motivators for some neurodiverse kids is that the pressure to earn praise or a reward can feel like yet another unpreferred task or demand on top of the unwanted thing they've been asked to do. Not only do they have to put on their pj's, but there is the additional pressure to earn that extra book or song. If this sounds like your child, the best motivators are *unplanned, unexpected* rewards that are given as close to the good behavior as possible. These should be tangible rewards, and not a promise of something later. And it goes without saying that the reward should be specific to your child and something they really, really like. Don't rely on those same tired old sticker charts. Families have described to me the following successful rewards: watching Kermit the Frog sing "Rainbow Connection" on a parent's phone, ripping up several sheets of paper, being able to do a superhero jump into Dad's arms, getting two Skittles, being swung around the room once, being shown five photos from a photo album, coloring a coloring sheet, or having a parent answer a fun question.

Finally, come up with several options, and have them ready. Unfortunately, rewards tend to lose their magic powers after about two weeks. Once one type of reward isn't so motivating anymore, you need to switch to something new that is.

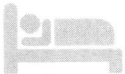

Tuck-In Tips

- Identify the underlying problem causing sleep issues, and set a realistic goal for improvement.
- Motivate your child to change their behavior using rewards. Coming up with good rewards is tricky. They work best when they are tangible and given immediately after the good behavior (and are not promises for later). Avoid rewards that might cause an epic meltdown if not earned,

and have several options, since rewards lose their magic over time.

- If the promise of a reward seems to increase your child's stress, only give surprise rewards they aren't expecting.

Pillow Point

Identify the problem with your neurodiverse child's sleep that most impacts the entire family, and make your goal taking achievable steps toward improving that problem.

Chapter 10

Communicate About Sleep

Neurodiverse people by nature see the world differently. We once took our kids to Disney World, and while walking to dinner at the hotel, Henry spontaneously ran into the elevator and pushed a button before we could get in with him or stop him. He got off the elevator wherever it stopped (there were many floors), and then he hid — most likely because he didn't understand what had happened or where he was.

I had no idea how to find him, and I became hysterical in the hotel lobby, begging the hotel manager for help. No words can express how powerless and terrified I felt. At home, Henry sometimes hid in the coat closet or under the table, and thanks to our wonderful behavior therapist Beth, we had taught Henry that if he heard us call, "Henry, where are you?" in a singsongy voice, he would respond, "Here I am!" We had practiced this quite a lot at home, so through my tears, I tried to singsong-scream for him. Henry's dad visited different floors while I stayed in the lobby yelling. After the longest fifteen minutes of my life, a little voice called out, "Here I am, Mommy."

That evening, our guardian-angel hotel manager sent a gift basket to our room as an extra treat. After bedtime, while stress-eating Mickey Mouse–shaped Rice Krispy treats, I tried to put myself in Henry's shoes. Why had he done that? I realized he had no clue that when you push the number button in an elevator, it goes to that floor. He had no idea that hotels have different floors. He didn't understand that when you get in an elevator and push the button, you don't always get to see Mickey Mouse. Why hadn't I taught him about elevators? Neurodiverse kids don't always perceive things the way we expect or as others do; that's part of what makes them wonderfully different. They may not intuitively pick up expectations or watch other people to figure out how something works, so they need someone to break it down and communicate the steps explicitly. This is true about sleeping. To most people, sleeping is simple: You get ready for bed, get into the bed, turn the light off, and go to sleep. Then you stay asleep in your bed until you wake up in the morning. To some people, this process is a mystery, and each step must be taught.

If you haven't done so before, make sure to communicate to your neurodiverse child what sleep entails, breaking it down into specific steps and clear behaviors. The whole process of getting to sleep involves several transitions, all of which can be challenging for neurodiverse kids.

1. Stop the current activity, which may be preferred.
2. Start a new activity (the bedtime routine), which is likely not preferred.
3. At the end of the routine, get into bed and turn the lights off.
4. While in bed, the body is still, the voice is quiet, and (usually) the eyes are closed.
5. Then wait for sleep to arrive and stay asleep (or remain quiet and safe in bed) until morning.

How you phrase these steps is up to you and what works best for your child. I suggest using simple instructions that emphasize the desired action or behavior ("body is still" rather than "stop moving"). In addition, I like to use the phrase "wait for sleep" rather than "try to go to sleep." The reason is that any effort to make sleep happen usually gets in the way. Framing this as "waiting" versus "trying" might alleviate a bit of anxiety, and it sets up a realistic expectation about falling asleep.

Visual Aids, Charts, Checklists, and Stories

To teach neurodiverse kids about expectations, situations, and desired behaviors, therapists of all types, teachers, paraprofessionals, and other experts have developed several effective communication methods, in various modalities, including assistive communication devices. The main ones are "first/then" visual aids, charts, checklists, and social stories, which I describe below. While these work consistently for many neurodiverse people, consider your child's age, developmental level, and preferred method of communication. It can be helpful to ask the professionals on your child's team the best ways they've found to communicate to children with similar needs and neurodiversity. I also try to use simple, memorable language. For example, they know the areas they must wash every time they get in the tub: face and hands, pits (armpits), piggies (toes and feet), and privates. They think the three P's are funny, and it's been easy for them to remember.

Examples of visual aids, charts, and social stories related to bedtime and sleep can be found on my website (www.drmelisa moore.com). Feel free to use these or modify them for your child. In addition, you can find examples on the internet that cover thousands of different scenarios.

First/Then Visuals

The first/then or when/then concept is to create a visual that represents two actions, one a result of the other. If the child does something *first*, or *when* they do it, *then* they get to do the other thing. Typically, the other thing is a reward, or something the child prefers. Visually, this is usually represented by two illustrations or pictures, each labeled, on either side of a rectangle divided in half. The left side is red and is the "first/when" task; the right side is green and is the "then" reward. For example, at bedtime, if you want to convey to your child that they must take a shower before reading books, it might look like this:

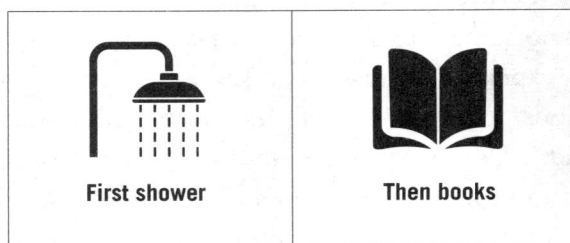

| First shower | Then books |

Introduce the first/then card just before the shower — or anytime your child asks for the reward during other parts of the routine. It can help to keep a few cards in different spots around the house so they're easy to grab when you need them. For example, if your child asks for a book during their bedtime snack, you can show them the first/then card you've tucked away in the kitchen. It may take several tries for your child to grasp the first/then concept, so keep it light and consistent.

Bedtime Chart

Bedtime charts are visual representations of the sequence of steps in the bedtime routine. These can increase predictability and decrease anxiety at bedtime. The visuals can be clip art, stick figure drawings, or pictures from online, and words are optional. While it's good if the pictures correspond to your child and setting, the details do not have to exactly correspond. For example, it's fine to use a picture of a blue bathtub, even if yours is white. I recommend creating a chart that makes it easy to print multiples. Post the bedtime chart in the room where the child sleeps, and at the very beginning of the bedtime routine, review all the steps. You can point to each step and name it. You may also want to put one copy in the bathroom and/or other locations where the routine occurs. So, when your child asks for another book, you can point to the chart and say, "Look, the chart says we only read three books." Below is an example.

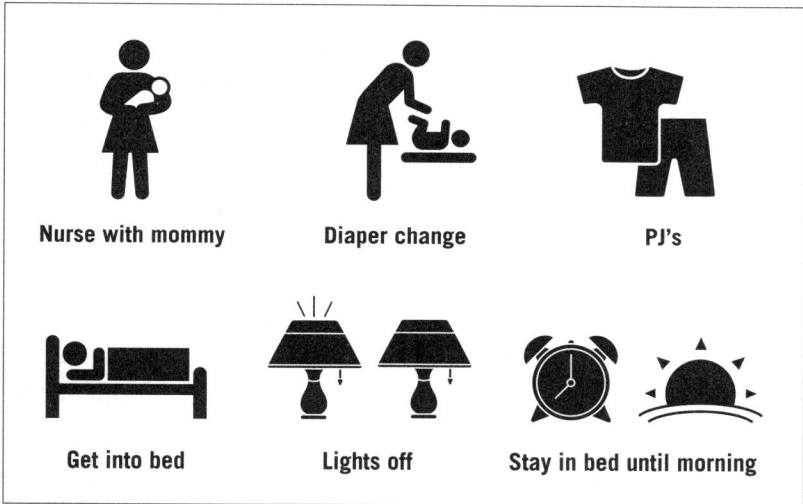

Nurse with mommy	Diaper change	PJ's
Get into bed	Lights off	Stay in bed until morning

Bedtime Checklist

Checklists are another simple way to help neurodiverse kids of all ages get things done. They can also be good tools for facilitating independence. You can use a dry-erase board or a laminated, wipe-off chart, or use Velcro-backed pictures or words that start on the left and that are moved to the right when the task is complete. The checklist could be in pictures rather than words or on your child's assistive communication device. As your child is learning, review the whole list at the beginning of the routine, before each individual step, and/or at the end of the routine to make sure everything has been completed. Once they understand it, you can simply review their completed checklist when they report that they are done.

Here is an example of a simple checklist that uses words.

Bedtime Checklist	
Sit on toilet. Wipe, flush, and wash hands.	
Shower: Wash face, hands, pits, piggies, and privates. Dry off.	
Put on clean undies and pj's.	
Brush teeth.	
Put dirty clothes in hamper.	
Bring three books to Mom's bed.	

As I discuss in chapter 13, treating the chart or checklist like a game can improve cooperation with the bedtime routine. Visual timers are a great way to show how much time has passed. There are simple, analog visual timers as well as apps with cool timers that slowly reveal a picture. If your child has difficulty finishing their bedtime routine in a timely way, make it a goal to finish the steps in thirty minutes (with or without your help). When the timer goes off, if they are done, clap and cheer and perhaps offer a reward like an extra book, video clip, or joke. If they haven't finished in time, reinforce what they've done, but do not give the extra reward.

When Henry was a toddler, I repurposed a monster truck race–themed board game from the dollar store. I wrote the steps in the bedtime routine along the route and added Velcro squares to the back of the game pieces. As each step was completed, Henry moved the game piece forward until he reached the finish line. He was so distracted by the game that he forgot it was bedtime! Now, that's the sort of bedtime game you want your child to play.

Social Stories

Social stories are one of the most common methods of conveying information and expectations about a variety of situations to neurodiverse kids. Social stories were developed in the early 1990s by Carol Gray for children with ASD.[1] However, I've found them to be helpful for almost all children. Social stories have evolved over time, yet the purpose and components have stayed the same. Here are the steps to make your own:

1. Determine the situation or behavior you want to highlight. Be specific.
2. Identify potential challenges.
3. Write simple, short sentences, describing sequence, expectations, and positive outcomes.
4. Add visuals and personalize it.

Social stories are typically written either in first person or third person. That is, either they read as if the child is speaking, using "I," or they read as if they are about the child, using their name and appropriate pronouns. There are usually simple images that accompany each sentence in the story, which can be repeated throughout. Each sentence and image are on a separate page or a different line, as shown in the example on the next page.

Social stories convey information. The goal is to describe the situation and order of events, give direction, connect to the child's feelings, affirm the positive, and highlight who and what can be helpful in the situation. The parent or child reads the story out loud in advance to prepare for unfamiliar situations like going on an airplane or starting a new school. When it comes to sleep, I suggest reading the story once or twice each night before starting the bedtime routine. Once the child understands the expectations around sleep, you no longer need to read the social story.

The following example is a social story about sleep, written in first person.

My Sleep Story

Sleep helps my brain and body rest and be happy and healthy.

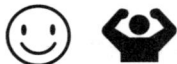

To get ready for bed, I have to stop what I am doing and start my bedtime routine.

If I don't want to stop and I feel sad or mad, I will still be OK.

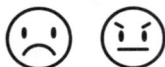

I can play again tomorrow.

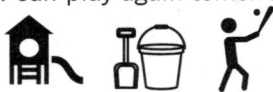

First, I have a snack at the kitchen table.

Then I go upstairs and sit on the toilet.

I wash my hands.

Then I brush my teeth.

Next, I put on clean pj's.

I go to my mom's room and we read three books.

Then I go to my room. I get into my bed with my dog stuffie.

When I am ready, Mom gives me a hug, turns off the light, and shuts the door.

If I don't feel tired, that is OK! I wait quietly in my bed with my eyes closed.

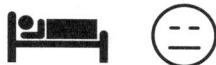

I stay in my bed all night. If there is an emergency or I feel sick, I will wake Mom.

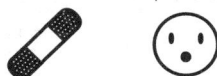

When I see that my morning light is on, it is OK to get up!

When I get a good night's sleep I am happy, rested, and ready to have fun today!

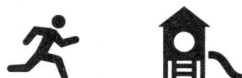

Other Communication Methods

For younger children, those with visual or auditory impairment, or those who respond better to touch, try the hand-over-hand technique to teach the bedtime routine. This simply means that you put your hand over your child's as you help them do the step. For example, you put your hand over theirs and gently guide them to brush their own teeth or wash their own face. For those who aren't auditory learners, light taps on the arm can give a countdown or be an indicator for the next step. You might say or sign, "When I give you three taps, I'm going to rinse your hair. Ready? One, two, three, go."

When it comes to helping children understand when it's morning, or when they can get out of bed, I *don't* recommend relying on the clock or the sun. If you teach, "When it's dark out, it's time to sleep," that can backfire — such as during the summer when bedtime is 7:30 p.m., but it's not dark until 9 p.m.

One way to help children understand when it is OK to get out of bed is to use a morning light (as opposed to a nightlight) that turns on or changes color at a certain time. There are a million versions of this on the market, or you can just put a regular nightlight on a timer to turn *on* in the morning. The nightlight's purpose is to slightly illuminate the room, while the morning light is a cue that it's OK to get out of bed. This light shouldn't be bright enough to wake your child, but they should be able to see it from their bed.

Even if your child is a pro at telling time, the simplicity of light on/light off works better than a clock. For all people, clock watching usually makes insomnia worse. I like to have the light turn *on* sometime between 5 a.m. and 7 a.m. If the problem is that your child wakes up too early, you want to start with success, so initially set it for the earliest reasonable time for you. Once your child understands what the morning light means, you can gradually move wake time later by fifteen minutes every day or so until you reach your ideal time.

If your child cannot perceive light, you can replace the morning light with a morning sound. If your child already uses a sound machine, pick one with a different sound to come *on* when it is OK to get out of bed. Make it just loud enough for your child to hear but not so loud it wakes them up.

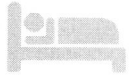

Tuck-In Tips

- Neurodiverse kids don't always inherently understand sleep expectations, and they may need to be taught the steps for getting ready for bed, going to sleep, staying in bed, and waking up.
- Visual aids, social stories, charts, and checklists are effective modes of communication to teach neurodiverse children about sleep.
- A morning light or morning sound is better than a clock or the sun for cueing your child that it is OK to get out of bed.

Pillow Point

It's key to communicate the steps involved in getting ready for bed and the expectations around sleep, doing so in the way your child learns best.

Chapter 11

Open the Door for Sleep (aka the Dreaded Sleep Hygiene)

I saw a new family recently, and they started the visit by saying, "Please, no more sleep hygiene." Their eight-year-old daughter Jane also requested "no breathing." This made me laugh and reminded me of another time I was asked for no breathing. My younger son, Simon, came into my room several years ago and asked to get into my bed because he'd had a bad dream. He snuggled in, and after only one of us fell asleep, I woke up to his voice: "Hey, Mommy? Mommy? Can you please stop making that sound?"

I had no idea what he was talking about. "What sound?" I asked. "Was I snoring?"

"No, it's just that air sound you make." I kissed his head and told him to go back to sleep, but he was persistent. "Mommy, I can't sleep when you are making that in and out air sound."

I laughed. "Honey, I'm just breathing."

He asked earnestly, "Well, then can you please stop breathing?"

Sleep hygiene refers to establishing consistent sleep habits that promote a full night's sleep (appropriate to the person's age). Sleep hygiene is important, but establishing an "ideal" routine with a neurodiverse child can be virtually impossible. Further, providers sometimes present sleep hygiene like a cure-all that parents must not have heard of before. In this family's case, Jane and her father both had ADHD and difficulty falling asleep, and they knew all about sleep hygiene.

Jane's parents told me about a recent psychiatry appointment where they were asked about their daughter's sleep. At first, they were happily surprised that finally someone had even asked about it, as it had always been challenging. Jane's mom described all the steps in her daughter's bedtime routine, which led to a daily bedtime at 10 p.m. or so and a wake time of 6 a.m. or so. The psychiatrist immediately identified Jane's less-than-ideal sleep hygiene as the reason for her sleep problems, and he focused on why her daughter ate a bedtime snack *after* she brushed her teeth. This psychiatrist thought the cure for Jane's ADHD-related sleep problems was as simple as improving sleep hygiene. As Socrates said, "You don't know what you don't know."

Jane's mom told me she felt like she was a kid in trouble for forgetting to do her homework. Did this psychiatrist really think that she didn't know they had a less-than-ideal bedtime routine? She said her blood was starting to boil and she was ready to tell him off. Instead, she pretended to be an actress playing the part of Jane's mom, so that she could keep her cool. As she described it, in scene one, her character calmly explained the situation, even smiling sometimes and slipping in an "as you know," while silently screaming inside. Their family had tried various bedtimes throughout the years, but when Jane got into bed earlier than about 10 p.m., she took another one to three hours to fall asleep. On the nights she didn't fall asleep quickly, her brain tended to blast off with exciting new Minecraft ideas or worries about the next day, and she stayed awake even later.

In scene two, Jane's mom explained to the psychiatrist that teeth brushing often led to meltdowns that were so intense it took several hours for her daughter to regulate and calm down, which again led to her staying awake even later. And yet if she didn't have a snack at bedtime, she would wake up during the night yelling and hungry. Jane's mom ended her imaginary monologue not by quoting an ancient philosopher, but with equally profound words from rappers Busta and Biggie: "If you don't know, now you know." This play left me laughing in tears.

Parents of neurodiverse children and teens interact with a lot of providers. In our family's case, Henry's team at any given time might include a developmental pediatrician, endocrinologist, pulmonologist, occupational therapist, behavior therapist, speech therapist, and more. Whenever a new provider asks about my son's sleep, I get excited that sleep is on their radar, but when their recommendations are limited to "improve sleep hygiene," I deflate. In an ideal world, everyone who works with neurodiverse kids would consider sleep hygiene *and* also think about other factors that disrupt sleep.

But champions of sleep hygiene aren't wrong, either. However much, as parents, we might want to throw good sleep hygiene out the window when it comes to our neurodiverse child, it is a necessary start to improving their sleep. As I discuss in chapter 2, a bedtime routine is like an invitation for sleep. This habitual sequence of events sets up an environment conducive to sleep, and it helps the brain and body "turn on" sleep and "turn off" wakefulness.

Because turning on sleep and turning off wakefulness are two distinct processes, I tackle them separately. In chapter 12, I discuss strategies for calming wakefulness, and in this chapter, I discuss setting up sleep-promoting conditions.

The Superpowers of a Bedtime Routine

A bedtime routine is critical when it comes to setting the stage for sleep.[1] Depending on what's included, a bedtime routine can promote multiple areas of well-being: nutrition (bedtime snack), hygiene, toileting, fine motor skills, reading, joint attention (anything done together), executive functioning (planning for the next day), behavior and emotion regulation (engaging in nonpreferred or anxiety-provoking activities), and cultivating independence. In addition to that hotbed of benefits, a bedtime routine is the first step in turning on sleep. Sometimes parents worry if their child starts fussing as soon as they realize the bedtime routine is starting, but this is actually a good thing. It means that the brain is making the association between the routine and sleep, which we want. It's hard to recommend exactly what your child's bedtime routine should include because it will be specific to your family. But here are five general tips:

The Five S's of a Good Bedtime Routine

1. **Short:** Keep the routine to thirty to forty-five minutes, including a bath or shower.
2. **Sweet:** Right before bed, avoid tasks that your child really hates.
3. **Soothing:** Engage in a few calming activities, but do these outside of the bedroom or at least not in the bed. Avoid electronics if possible.
4. **Streamlined:** Start the routine outside of your child's bed or room (even reading and snuggling) and steadily move toward the place where the child will be sleeping. Once they are in bed, it's lights out, eyes closed, wait for sleep.
5. **Steady:** Keep all aspects of the environment — such as nightlights and sound machines — the same all night long.

The five S's are the ideal, so now let's meet up with the real. First, a consistent bedtime routine seven nights a week is ideal, but the benefits aren't all-or-nothing. Research shows that having a bedtime routine three nights is better than zero nights.[2] Stick to the routine as much as you can, and let it go when you can't. Next, get input (appropriate to their development) from your child when determining what the bedtime routine includes. All of us would prefer to avoid activities we don't like, and for neurodiverse children and teens, a typical bedtime routine includes challenging transitions and nonpreferred tasks. If possible, avoid activities that are especially difficult or typically lead to conflict. If your child takes medications they particularly hate, do that first, even before the bedtime snack. If they get upset with teeth brushing, consider a thorough brushing earlier in the evening, and at bedtime, do a quick once over. If independent reading is a big challenge, perhaps read to your child at bedtime instead of asking them to read.

Bedtime routines are also a great time to provide end-of-the-day sensory input. This might include anything from the joint compressions recommended by your child's occupational therapist to petting the cat for a few minutes. If it works for you, allow your child to choose from a list or a box of items that might appeal to their sense of smell or touch, such as scented room spray, a sequin pillow, a lavender sachet, a satin ribbon, a furry stuffed animal, a textured sticker, or an engaging fidget. In chapter 16, I discuss sensory sensitivities and sensory input in more detail, and in chapter 20, I describe what neurodivergent teenagers think about bedtime routines. Spoiler alert: They want a bespoke bedtime routine with custom sensory input.

Are Electronics Taboo?

Are electronics at bedtime the cause of the world's sleep problems? For almost a decade, I believed that screens — video games, TV, smartphones, social media, movies, and so on — were detrimental to sleep for everyone. That is, until I experienced the opposite.

For a period during kindergarten, Henry took two to three hours to fall asleep, and during this time he often quietly got out of bed to put on a superhero cape, play Legos, or color. Thank goodness he at least had a consistent bedtime routine and pretty good sleep hygiene, given that his mom was a sleep "expert." Per my usual recommendations to families, Henry got lots of sunlight and exercise, he ate meals at traditional mealtimes, and I took toys, books, and everything potentially entertaining out of his bedroom. Yet Henry still took forever to fall asleep, and he had a great time while he was waiting, enthralled by his very interesting fingers and amused by making shadows on the wall. It took even longer for him to fall asleep when I took toys and books out of his room because he got so silly. During that period, he snuck the iPad into his room a few times, and I caught him only because he was asleep within twenty minutes. To me that was confusing and didn't match the science I knew.

Sleep researchers found decades ago that the blue light from electronics temporarily stops the production of melatonin, the "sleep" hormone, and when blue light is taken away, melatonin turns back on again.[3] Theoretically, melatonin disruption in combination with the stimulating content of electronics — the game, show, video, and so on — should make it harder to fall asleep, and for many people it does. But as it turns out, this is not true for all people all the time.

One thing I love about science is that it evolves based on new research, which is what has happened with our understanding of the relationship between electronics and sleep. For over two decades, science told us that electronics harm sleep for everyone, and should be kept out of the bedroom.[4] In the summer of 2024, researchers from Sweden, Australia, and Israel published a paper summarizing findings from many high-quality studies and found that the impact of electronics on sleep depends on what the electronic device is, the content, who is using it, and how much they are using it, among other factors.[5] An alternate explanation for the relationship between electronics and trouble sleeping also emerged: People who already have trouble sleeping sometimes fill the time they are waiting for sleep with electronics. So are electronics the downfall of good sleep? It depends!

Sleep Environment

Along with creating a good bedtime routine, we also want to create the best sleep-promoting conditions we can. The best sleep environment is dark, cool, quiet, and comfortable. These factors have been studied in surprisingly specific detail, so we know exactly what is ideal for the average person's sleep.

Starting with temperature, you may have heard that the ideal setting for sleep is 65 to 68 degrees Fahrenheit. This has in fact been demonstrated in adults. Children tend to be more sensitive to temperature, and neurodiverse children may be the most sensitive of all. For a child, an ideal nighttime bedroom temperature is a few degrees warmer (70–73°F), and temperatures on either side of that range are associated with worse sleep.[6] It's not just the temperature of the room, either. According to a 2019 review of temperature-and-sleep research, a warm bath or shower within one to two hours of bedtime decreases the time it takes to fall asleep.[7] Warm water lowers body temperature, and lower body temperature promotes sleep. Of course, if your child hates getting wet, taking a warm bath an hour before sleep might be counterproductive, but the take-home message is that both ambient temperature and body temperature impact sleep.

Light also impacts sleep. It obviously helps to have a dark bedroom at night, but it's also important to have exposure to sunlight during the day. This is the main influence on our circadian rhythm. Not just any light will do. We need natural sunlight, especially in the morning, to keep our circadian clock on track. More, longer, and brighter sunlight is better, but don't worry, this doesn't mean your child has to go outside for hours in the winter as soon as the sun rises. Consider opening the shades in the morning and serving breakfast in a sunny place. In the evening, limit exposure to sunlight and electronics, and close those blackout shades.

Your child's room should also be quiet, and if you live in a creaky house like mine, a sound machine, fan, or air purifier can mask noises inside and outside the house. Jungle, ocean, crickets, train, white noise…it doesn't matter what the sound is as long as it covers up other nighttime sounds. Even small sounds that you may not notice can impact your neurodiverse child's sleep. For example, my son can hear a fly even outside of his room, and it destroys his sleep. There have been multiple times when I could be found at 2 a.m. running around the house with a fly swatter. Now for the sake of everyone's sleep, Henry's nightlight doubles as a plug-in bug deterrent. Win-win.

The fourth element of a good sleep environment is comfort. What does that mean? I've worked with a surprising number of parents who have purchased new bed frames, mattresses, sheets, and/or comforters in hopes that it will maximize their neurodiverse child's sleep. Guess what? I'm one of them, and I'm here to report from both a personal and professional perspective, none of that helps. Like many things, I judge comfort in terms of what promotes sleep, and especially for neurodiverse kids, "comfort" is unique to the individual. Is it long-sleeved pj's, no pj's, or sleeping in school clothes? Is it one blanket, a weighted blanked, or a stretchy Lycra sheet? Is it sleeping on the floor instead of in bed (even if parents feel guilty about it)? Do whatever is comfortable for your neurodiverse child, as long as it's safe. If your child is sleeping, you'll know they are comfortable enough.

WHEN TO TRANSITION TO A BIG KID BED

If your child is sleeping in a crib, do not move them to a toddler or big kid bed for as long as safely possible. Once they start climbing out of the crib, it's no longer safe, but delay the transition as long as you can. If another baby is on the way, borrow a crib or buy another one. I promise you won't regret it. Once your child is in a bed, they can easily get out, which makes learning to fall asleep independently much more difficult, especially for younger toddlers. At some point between ages three and five, children develop the cognitive ability to delay something they want. They are able to stay in bed, even if they don't want to in the moment. Most two-year-olds and some three- and four-year-olds can't do this, not because they are misbehaving, but because their brains don't work that way yet.

Get Ready for the Next Bedtime by Waking Up!

Believe it or not, preparation for nighttime sleep begins the moment we wake in the morning. This means having a consistent wake-up time, regardless of whether sleep was good or not-so-good the night before.

If it's a non-school day, your child should wake not more than two hours later than their school-day wake-up time. Though it might not always feel this way, it's biologically easier to wake up than it is to fall asleep. We can't force ourselves to fall asleep without medications or anesthesia, but most of us have forced ourselves to wake up when needed, for example, by standing up, taking a walk or a shower, drinking caffeine, or exercising. In general, pick a wake-up time that allows your child time to eat breakfast and get dressed, but not so much time that the process gets derailed by other activities. Do not build "snooze" time into wake-up time. Then get as much natural sunlight as possible in the morning. Have I said that already?

In addition to our brain's circadian cells, the circadian cells in our gastrointestinal system influence our body clock. Eating and drinking communicate to those cells that it's daytime. People ask me frequently what the best and worst foods are for sleep, and despite the rumors, there aren't consistent findings. Foods that affect your neurodiverse child's sleep are specific to them. The only exception is caffeine, which interferes with most everyone's sleep. Children should avoid caffeinated beverages in general, but especially after lunch. Caffeine has an alerting effect on children and teens, even if it's consumed with food at dinnertime. Caffeine is also often a "hidden" ingredient in vitamin waters, sweet teas, and fruity drinks, so check for it to avoid having a wild gremlin on your hands.

The sleep pressure we need to get to sleep at night builds during the day, so unless they are of napping age, kids and teens should avoid all daytime sleep. This might be difficult for a sleepy adolescent, but I promise you it is not impossible. The body's circadian rhythm naturally dips briefly in the afternoon around 3 p.m., and a bit of sleepiness is common. If your child is sleepy after school, encourage activities that are incompatible with sleep, such as going for a bike or a scooter ride, playing a game, or talking to a friend. A thirty-minute electronics break or a quick run around the block can get your child or teen over that afternoon slump.

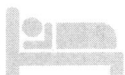

Tuck-In Tips

- Healthy sleep hygiene is necessary, but it is not always sufficient for a good night's sleep, especially in neurodiverse children and teens.
- Start with a regular bedtime and wake-up time on school days. On non-school days, keep wake-up time within two hours of the regular time.
- Turning sleep on and wakefulness off are two separate processes, and both are helped with a consistent bedtime routine.
- Create a bedtime routine based on the five S's: short, sweet, soothing, streamlined, steady.
- Keep the sleeping space cool, dark, quiet, and comfortable.
- Get as much natural sunlight in the morning as possible and eat at traditional mealtimes.
- Do not sleep during the day unless a nap is age appropriate.

Pillow Point

For healthy sleep hygiene, maintain a consistent sleep schedule, have a bedtime routine as many days per week as possible, get sunlight exposure in the morning, and avoid daytime napping.

Chapter 12

Waiting for Sleep to Arrive

After a very consistent bedtime routine, one family I worked with had an especially challenging time getting their neuro-diverse teen to the finish line. Fourteen-year-old Layla had ASD, schizophrenia, and insomnia. When it was time for lights out, Layla repeatedly got in and out of bed and paced in her room or in the hall for hours becoming increasingly tired and frustrated. Once she was calm enough to stay in her bed for ten to fifteen minutes, Layla fell asleep quickly and easily. Layla's parents knew that sleep was near when Layla stayed in bed for longer than ten minutes. After hearing this, I knew we had to get creative to help Layla stay in her bed once the lights were turned off.

Layla especially enjoyed tearing up pieces of butcher paper or newspaper, throwing cards from a deck one by one on the floor, watching Beyoncé and Rihanna music videos, looking at pictures of family members on a phone, and playing with a few different fidgets. The family didn't want to use ripping paper or throwing cards at bedtime, as those were incentives for other important daytime behaviors. Our unconventional first step was for Layla to watch her favorite videos in bed immediately after her bedtime routine. This was nowhere near ideal, but we had to think outside the box. After about two weeks of this, Layla stayed in her bed watching videos for ten to fifteen minutes and fell asleep quickly once the lights were off. While it was awesome she was staying in her bed, we had also created a sleep association that wasn't helpful.

Though Layla was awake enough to put down the iPad when the timer went off after ten minutes, she relied on those videos to calm down enough for sleep. Because we had replaced the walking/sleep association with the iPad/sleep association, Layla continued to wake two to three times during the night yelling for Mom and Grandma. She became agitated to the point of hitting herself until her mom or grandma showed Layla videos or family photographs on their phones. Eventually, Layla fell back to sleep.

We took a step back and moved bedtime thirty minutes earlier to ensure that Layla was wide awake after her bedtime routine, so she could learn to soothe herself. We allowed her to keep watching videos of Beyoncé ("Single Ladies") and Rihanna ("Umbrella"), but we kept the lights on and had her sit on top of the covers. When those two videos were over, lights were turned off, and Layla got under the covers to fall asleep on her own. We found the sweet spot where Layla was calm enough to stay in her bed but awake enough to soothe herself to sleep on her own in twenty to thirty minutes. However, she still experienced one long waking of one to two hours during the night, and Layla's mom and grandma were exhausted and frankly sick of looking at pictures of themselves in the middle of the night. We brainstormed more and decided to print several of Layla's favorite family photographs and put them in a soft, cloth photo album. Eventually, Layla learned to stay quietly in her bed looking at the album until she returned to sleep on her own, which was enormous progress.

Finding the Sweet Spot of Calming Distraction

After the bedtime routine, once your neurodiverse child has made it to their bed, the goal is for them to stay calm and wait for sleep to arrive. It is normal to take ten to thirty minutes to fall asleep, even if it feels like an eternity. In fact, falling asleep within minutes is a sure sign of sleep deprivation. Once we are snug in our beds with lights off and eyes closed, all we can do is wait. For neurodiverse kids and teens, this is when the right amount of distraction is key.

I came to this conclusion after working with several wonderful families where ADHD was in the mix. It started with an eleven-year-old, nonbinary child named Cody with severe ADHD. Cody's father was forthright about his own ADHD, and he dove right into his child's appointment by telling me about his own bedtime routine. To fall asleep easily, Cody's dad either needed *The Great British Baking Show* on in the background or he had to use "thinking games," such as repeating the numbers in the Fibonacci sequence (a series where each number is the sum of the two numbers before it: 1, 2, 3, 5, 8, 13, 21…), which is not a terrible idea, given that the Fibonacci sequence is infinite. He wanted to figure out what equivalent tricks might work for Cody. This was another aha moment for me.

We typically view distraction, inattention, and lack of focus as negative, but when it comes to sleep, they can be downright helpful for neurodivergent people. While waiting for sleep to arrive, the goal is for the brain to be calm but occupied to the extent that internal thoughts and ideas don't steamroll sleep. When I discussed this idea with lauded ADHD expert Dr. Kathleen Nadeau, she hypothesized that the perfect level of distraction quiets the default mode network (for more on this, see chapter 4), which is often too active at bedtime to welcome sleep. A relaxed and perfectly distracted mind is ready for sleep.

Another potential barrier to sleep during this vulnerable time of waiting is mood. Neurodiverse children and teens are at increased risk of mood disorders, and lying still in a dark, quiet room at night is prime time for anxious and depressing thoughts and feelings to emerge. When kids are anxious and/or depressed, especially in times of acute distress, I emphasize both distraction and connection. If possible, help your child identify effective ways to keep their mind occupied and relaxed, even if it is via an audiobook, music, or a show. Again, a relaxed and occupied mind leaves little space for ruminating on the past or the future, and it turns focus away from unhelpful thoughts and worries at night. This does not mean ignoring or teaching your child to avoid difficult feelings. Check in about their day, their mood, their worries, and other tough topics a few hours before bedtime. Most teenagers want to be alone when falling asleep, but if you can, stay aware and connected in some way during that vulnerable time when they're waiting for sleep.

I like to ask people what they do while they wait for sleep, which is a weird icebreaker. Dr. Ali Downes, our developmental pediatrician, said that she counts backward from one hundred by sevens. I work with a little girl who loves math, and she goes through her multiplication facts. A boy who loves Disneyland imagines each ride in detail. I like to strategize with families to figure out realistic, quiet, effective ways to wait for sleep, and then we make reminder cards to put on a ring and take home. These might include ways of breathing, muscle relaxation, imagery, fidgets, math sequences, remembering dialogue from movies, chronicling events, and thinking about specific characteristics of people or places. It might involve reviewing all the details of favorite objects, like lawn mowers or steam trains. There are tricks for keeping your mind busy, such as the cognitive shuffle, where you start with a word like *bedtime* and think of everything you can that starts with each letter.[1] For *B*, words might include *banana*, *boat*, *bird*, and so on, and you picture each thing in your mind as you go along. Or think of everything you can for each color of the rainbow — for red, that might be *apple*, *fire truck*, *strawberry*, *stop sign*, and so on — while picturing each one in your mind.

There are infinite ways that people calm down to sleep, and unfortunately some are loud and can even be unsafe. Some children or teens will rock back and forth or bang their heads to transition to sleep. You did not cause this; it is an association that develops on its own and isn't uncommon in neurodiverse children. As I mention in chapter 5, you can move the crib or bed to the middle of the room, put a mattress on the floor, or co-sleep, but it's still a tough one to eliminate. There isn't a foolproof way to stop it. So identify the specific problem. Do the rocking and banging wake up the whole house? Is the movement scraping the floor? Those have solutions, which may not involve changes to sleep. If your child or teen is hurting themselves, this is serious and warrants a visit with a developmental pediatrician, neurologist, or other trusted member of your team.

Tuck-In Tips

- A calm yet distracted mind is best while waiting for sleep. Help your child identify ways to stay relaxed and occupied, which may take significant trial and error.
- Falling asleep without medication typically takes ten to thirty minutes. If it only takes a minute or two, that's a sign of sleep deprivation.
- Depressive and anxious thoughts and feelings often surface when it is time for sleep. Talk about these feelings with your child long before bedtime.

Pillow Point

For neurodiverse kids, it's helpful to find strategies that both calm and occupy the mind while waiting for sleep to arrive, which should take about ten to thirty minutes.

Chapter 13

Bedtime Conflicts and Positive Sleep Associations

Bedtime problems like stalling, acting out, and/or needing a parent to fall asleep can get in the way of efficiently falling asleep and cause many parents to dread this time of night. I can relate, not because of bedtime, but because I dread dinnertime. I used to love to cook, but now dinner is an ever-present thorn in my side. My friends and I often text each other surprised and annoyed: "Are you kidding me? Is it really time to make dinner *again*?" Although I love spending time with my kids, dinner is tricky. One day a week I work late, and a huge benefit, to me, is that I get to miss making dinner. I mean, who wouldn't want to avoid the grind of meal planning, grocery shopping, and cooking dinner only to be met by a litany of complaints and the question, "Why is everything you make yucky?" My husband has largely taken over making dinner for the past year because of my work schedule, and guess what? I still dread it when it's my night to cook.

Just like avoiding dinner, avoiding bedtime isn't really a sustainable strategy, so this chapter provides advice for coping with bedtime resistance, complaints, and conflicts, as well as recommendations for establishing positive sleep associations.

Coping with Bedtime Conflicts

Sometimes for neurodiverse kids and teens, bedtime is the first time they've slowed down enough to think about the homework they were supposed to finish or the library book due tomorrow or the kid who tripped them in gym class. These thoughts can lead to big feelings, which can lead to bedtime problems. To stave off those bedtime realizations — and yet still talk about difficult feelings and situations — establish a check-in time or a "worry time" at a point in the day other than bedtime. Before the bedtime routine starts, have your child (with appropriate help) pack their backpack, pick out their clothes, and do any other tasks needed to get ready for the following day. As an aside: If getting dressed in the morning is a struggle, consider having your child change into tomorrow's clothes at bedtime and sleep in them. Many neurodiverse kids do this, and it can be a game changer.

With next-day preparations covered, include the last-minute things your child typically asks for as a regular part of the bedtime routine. If they frequently ask for water as you're turning off the lights, then a drink of water can be one of the last steps before getting into bed. Depict the steps and communicate any changes in the bedtime routine on a bedtime chart or a bedtime checklist (see chapter 10).

If the routine is a struggle, try to preempt negative behaviors by making it a game. Maybe set a timer for fifteen minutes, and if the bedtime checklist is finished when the timer goes off, there is a reward of an extra book or a short music video. As I describe in chapter 10, I once turned Henry's bedtime checklist into a board game that he became so engrossed playing he "forgot" he was actually getting ready for bed. Another option is to use a bedtime pass, which has scientifically been shown to reduce bedtime problems.[1] First, you and your child make and decorate paper passes together. Each pass can be traded for a short, reasonable request: a hug, a question, another tuck in, and so on. An example is shown below.

★ BEDTIME PASS ★

Trade at bedtime for one:
Hug
Question
Tuck in
Drink of water
Fun fact

Or trade leftover passes at breakfast for:
Silver-dollar pancakes
Favorite cereal
15 minutes on iPad

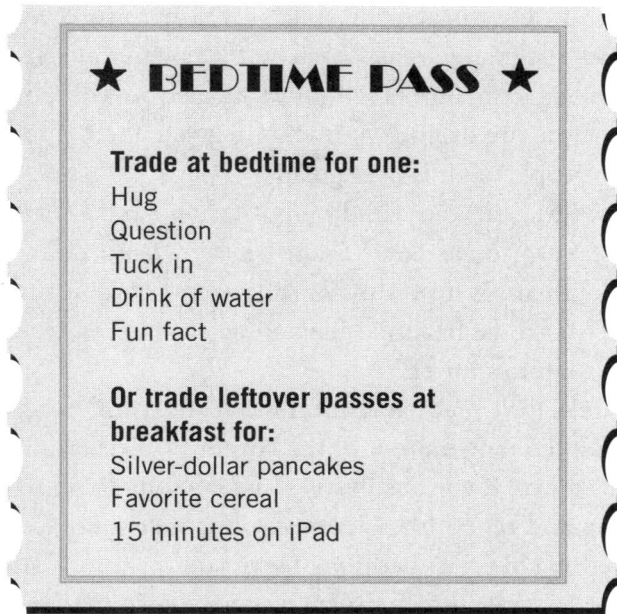

Decide how many passes to give during bedtime; usually three is a good number to start. The child can trade the pass for a reasonable request, which is granted. Once the passes are all used, parents no longer respond to requests (with the exception of safety or illness).

I recommend trying this for three to seven days until your child gets used to the system. Once they understand it and you think they can be successful, give a reward in the morning for any passes that are left over. Rewards should be small but motivating — I've seen families offer whipped cream on waffles, a special cereal, ten minutes of screen time, a game of twenty questions, and so on. Gradually reduce the number of passes from three to one.

Unfortunately, despite every attempt to prevent it, sometimes bedtime devolves into a cesspool of conflict. And strong emotions = high cortisol = wide awake. When there is no way to avoid a meltdown or tantrum, I approach it in one of four ways. I've tried to come up with a clever acronym for this, but *JMIS* is the best I can do.

1. **Join:** Sit down near your child, speaking only if needed and in a soothing voice. Focus on keeping yourself calm and taking long, slow breaths. By keeping yourself calm and steady, you are helping your child regulate their emotions. Some people call this co-regulation.

2. **Match:** Match your child's emotion and reflect it back, then commiserate. Say: "*I hate showers, too!* I don't want to take them! It makes me *so* sad when I have to stop my show. But to be healthy I have to be clean, even though I don't want to shower."

3. **Ignore:** Don't react and continue to do your thing, observing the tantrum out of the corner of your eye until it winds down. If you absolutely must say something, keep it boring and repetitive. Channel your inner robot and say something like, "It's bedtime. I love you."

4. **Space:** Separate for a moment by going to a different room or to the other side of the room, giving you both space to calm down. This is especially good for teenagers and gives them an escape hatch. At a time other than bedtime, discuss the benefits of taking space. Taking a little time away from the upsetting situation is one way to stop the spark from becoming a bonfire. Encourage your child to ask for space on their own so they can sidestep any aggression or acting out (and the consequences).

As discussed in chapter 9, it's most effective to give rewards and consequences as close to the positive behavior as possible; however, when it comes to sleep, this isn't always productive. To minimize bedtime struggles, I suggest delaying tough conversations and largely postponing rewards and consequences until the next day. Try to keep your own temperature down with calm, slow breathing and by focusing on your senses, staying in the present, and telling yourself something both positive and true. Examples are: "I've made it through thousands of bedtimes already, and I'll get through this one," or "She always falls asleep, even when it takes a while."

Changing Problematic Sleep Associations

In addition to coping with bedtime problems, managing problematic sleep associations — also called cues, connections, or signals — is essential. Why would parents want to change sleep associations in the first place? The most common reason is that they want to reduce their child's night wakings. Remember: Whatever sleep associations are needed at bedtime to calm down and to fall asleep will be needed to independently and easily return to sleep during the normal night wakings that are part of a sleep cycle. Another reason to manage sleep associations is that parents may need or want grown-up time to decompress rather than spending hours helping their child fall asleep. They might not want their bedtime to be the same as their child's.

Sleep associations are not all inherently negative, and it's not necessary or possible to change all of them. A sound machine, stuffed animal, or special blanket are all positive sleep associations: They promote self-soothing to sleep. Sleep associations are negative when they are unwanted and/or involve another person. Note that I say *unwanted*, which is not the case with intentional co-sleeping. For instance, if a child associates going to sleep with being fed by bottle or breast, being rocked to sleep, or lying with a parent to fall asleep, that becomes negative when the person who is required to do those things is not OK with being the child's sleep association. Feeding, cuddling, and rocking can be special and foster connection with your child. While there is no need to give them up, the timing might need to be shifted so they are no longer intertwined with sleep. Move any potentially sleep-inducing elements to the very beginning of the bedtime routine. You could do ten minutes of rocking, then bath, pj's, and so on, making sure that your child is fully awake when lights go out.

When I recommend changing sleep associations at bedtime first, parents sometimes think I haven't understood their main difficulty, which is their child's night wakings. These parents don't necessarily have a problem with their bedtime routine, but they don't yet see the connection between bedtime and their child's inability to get back to sleep during the night. I'll say it again: If the child can't fall asleep without X at bedtime, they are unlikely to easily return to sleep without X during those normal night wakings.

Further, to keep the entire night from being a disaster, I also usually recommend not trying to change the night wakings until the child has learned to fall asleep completely on their own at their regular bedtime. At first, put 100 percent of your energy into how your child falls asleep the first time, changing whatever sleep associations need to be changed. Then when your child wakes during the night, do whatever you need to do in order for them (and everyone else in the house) to get back to sleep as quickly and easily as possible — even if that involves doing the exact things you are trying *not* to do at bedtime, like feeding or rocking to sleep.

Once a child can soothe themselves to sleep at bedtime for a few weeks, those skills tend to generalize to middle-of-the-night wakings and to naps. That said, while I typically suggest a gradual approach to changing sleep associations, an all-at-once approach is equally effective. One thing to consider is that while a gradual approach is often easier for parents, sometimes it's harder for kids. For some neurodiverse kids, any change is extremely upsetting. Twenty steps to gradually learn independent sleep skills is twenty changes. In that case, you may want to limit changes by skipping smaller steps and moving forward more quickly with fewer, bigger steps.

Here's how to change those sleep associations and say goodbye to night wakings.

For Those Who Take a Bottle or Breast at Bedtime

If you have an infant or toddler who breastfeeds or has a bottle at bedtime, tackle that as the first change in the bedtime routine. Babies get very relaxed and drowsy when they eat, and to learn how to soothe themselves to sleep without eating, they should be wide awake when they are put in their crib or bed. After feeding, go through whatever your routine is (bath, pj's, and so on), so they are wide awake again. Put your child into their crib or bed awake. You can pat or soothe them, you can sit somewhere just hanging out, or you can leave the room and monitor for safety and illness until they fall asleep, but let the child fall asleep without feeding. At any future wakings, you can feed them, just not at bedtime. Remember that these strategies are supported by more than fifty years of research, and there is no body of research demonstrating that this approach is harmful physically, emotionally, psychologically, or relationally.

If you think this will be a struggle for you or your child, start with a smaller step. Do the feeding and the routine, but instead of putting them right into the bed or crib, hold, rock, and/or pat them until they are asleep, and then transfer them to the bed or crib. After one to two weeks, or whenever you're ready, put your child down to sleep while they are awake, right after the routine, and follow the steps above.

For Those Who Feed During the Night

If your child is still feeding by bottle or breast during the middle of the night, that is the next thing to work on. You can start by reducing the amount of liquid in the bottle or the amount of time they are on the breast (which can be difficult) and/or you can also gradually eliminate one feeding at a time, which many pediatricians suggest. Keep in mind that when your baby wakes, they have no idea if it is 11 p.m. or 1 a.m. or 3 a.m., which means they don't know if this is the time they get to eat, and sometimes they fuss more. Gradually eliminating feedings works for some families, and if you can drop one feeding at a time and pat or rock your child back to sleep, go for it.

Sometimes a "dream feed" can stretch the time between wakings, and it saves you from worrying that your child is hungry. Just before you go to bed, pick your child up and try to feed them in their sleep. It is easier to do this with a bottle you can pop into their mouth than it is with a breast, and it doesn't always work. Regardless, the goal is to reduce your help during the night so your child can use the new sleep skills they've learned at bedtime.

For Those Who Need a Parent to Fall Asleep

Check out the sequence below. Depending on what everyone in your household can tolerate and how quickly you want to move this process along, start at the beginning, somewhere in the middle, or skip interim steps. If you want your child to fuss as little as possible, take smaller steps, knowing that the night wakings will likely continue until your child is falling asleep 100 percent independently. I recommend starting with a step where you're confident that your child will be able to stay in bed until they fall asleep. So, if you've been lying in bed with them until they fall asleep, and one night you give them a tuck in and walk out, they will likely get out of bed to follow you. Instead, step-by-step, adjust your position relative to your child — in their bed and in the room — until you can walk out without being followed. Overall, minimize eye contact, talking, and other attention once lights are out. Continue with the same step for a few nights until your child is falling asleep at bedtime within about thirty minutes — or whenever you're ready to move on to the next step. Keep in mind that at every step, the goal is for your child to stay in their bed at bedtime until they fall asleep.

Here's one possible sequence for a parent who is currently lying in their child's bed until the child falls asleep.

1. Lie in bed beside your child, and reduce snuggling, hand-holding, or other physical contact.
2. Lie in bed beside your child without physical contact. Gently redirect your child's hands away if needed.
3. Sit up in bed beside your child, without physical contact.
4. Sit on the bed, without physical contact.
5. Sit beside the bed, and only if needed, place a hand on their back, hold their hand, or gently pat.
6. Sit closer to the door, without physical contact.
7. Take short breaks and leave the room. Say that you're leaving, and name a task, not a time: "Mom needs to change her clothes," "Dad needs to grab his phone." Don't say, "I'll be back in ten minutes," or you risk creating a clock-checking fanatic. Initially, leave only for a few seconds, or as long as you think your child will stay in bed. Every few nights, gradually increase the length of time you are gone.
8. Once your child is falling asleep on their own during the breaks, switch to leaving right away, and then returning to check on them. After lights out, say something like, "I'm going to do the dishes and then I'll check on you," or "I'm going to let the dog out and then I'll check on you." Leave only for as long as you think your child will stay in bed. When you do check, limit it to a quick peek. Sometimes kids try to stay awake for the check, but if they briefly fall asleep and miss it, they might wake and think no one has checked. It helps to anticipate this, and when you do

your check, put a blank sticky note on the door where they can see it. If they wake, they'll know you checked just like you promised.

Once your child falls asleep at bedtime, regardless of what step you're on, this part of the process is done. Be consistent and move forward at your own pace, helping your child learn to fall asleep at bedtime on their own. In the meantime, if your child wakes during the night, just do whatever is necessary to get them back to sleep. Once they have the skills to fall asleep 100 percent independently at bedtime, it can take one to three weeks for those skills to generalize to the rest of the night. At that stage, parents often don't hear about the night wakings anymore because their little one can get back to sleep on their own.

Fading Night Wakings

If your child now falls asleep on their own and you don't hear from them until morning, awesome! You don't need to do the next steps. Or if you don't mind that your child comes into your bed in the middle of the night or you are OK with being woken during the night for another tuck in, you also can skip this part. Otherwise, when you're ready, move to the next phase: Keep them in the crib or bed when they wake during the night.

Two to three weeks after your child can fall asleep 100 percent independently, repeat the process you used at bedtime, and gradually reduce your presence during the night (see also chapter 14). If you prefer a faster (yet arguably more challenging) approach, when your child wakes during the night and cries out, allow them to get back to sleep without you. Quickly and silently peek at your child at regular intervals or use a baby monitor to check for safety or illness. Occasionally those chubby toddler thighs get stuck between the crib slats. Other than monitoring your child, let the child figure out how to get back to sleep on their own.

When you do respond to a night waking, you might pat their back or rub their tummy and say something short and sweet: "It's sleep time. I love you." But try to leave them in their bed or crib without picking them up. Over time, reduce the patting and talking each night until they can return to sleep without your help. If you absolutely *must* pick them up, briefly settle them down, give a quick hug and put them right back into their crib or bed *awake*. I've frequently seen babies and toddlers get more upset after being picked up and put back down, so do what works for you and your child.

Naps

Naps tend to be a moving target. The need for naps changes with development, naps often occur outside the home, and if your child is in daycare or preschool, they are surrounded by peers who are also napping. While it's a good idea to try to be consistent, don't worry if naps sometimes vary.

Naps are a great time to practice those self-soothing skills your child has learned at night: tucking themselves in, keeping the brain calm and busy while waiting for sleep, and using a special sign to connect to a parent. A sweet example of a special sign is described in the book *The Kissing Hand* by Audrey Penn, where a hand on the cheek is a reminder of the mom's love.

Most of the time kids fall asleep at naptime more easily using the same sleep associations they use at night, so if you've tackled bedtime and middle of the night wakings, you probably have already tackled naps. In any case, at naptime, do a very brief version of the bedtime routine. That could be: Read one book, put on the sleep sack, and turn on the sound machine. If naps are still problematic, and your child is currently taking *two naps*, start working on the first one and leave the second one as is until the first nap is better. In other words, treat the first nap like bedtime and the second nap like a middle-of-the-night waking. If your child is currently taking *one nap*, put them in their bed or crib and allow them to fall asleep on their own. If after thirty to forty-five minutes they are still awake, take them out of their bed and do a quick activity, such as a walk around the block or playtime with a toy. Then try the nap again about fifteen to thirty minutes later. On days when naps are less than ideal, move bedtime earlier by about thirty minutes.

If, after you follow these steps, middle-of-the-night and early-morning wakings continue to be problematic, read the next chapter.

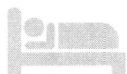

Tuck-In Tips

- Include your child's most frequent last-minute requests like a hug or sip of water as a regular part of the bedtime routine.
- Avoid bedtime battles when possible. Follow the JMIS strategy: join, match, ignore, space.
- If you want to reduce problematic night wakings, start with bedtime and change any sleep associations that require an adult's presence. Gradually lessen your involvement until your child can fall asleep independently.
- For children who are fed to sleep by breast or bottle, make the nighttime feeding the first step of the bedtime routine. Then make sure your child is fully awake when they are put down to sleep.
- Once your child has gone from wide awake to calm to asleep 100 percent independently at bedtime for at least two weeks, those skills often transfer to the middle of the night. If they don't, then fade yourself directly from night wakings and then from naps.

- If change is especially difficult for your child, move forward in fewer (and possibly bigger) steps.

Pillow Point

The key to your child easily falling asleep and returning to sleep on their own during normal night wakings is to (1) reduce bedtime problems and (2) help them learn to fall asleep on their own at bedtime.

Chapter 14

Persistent Middle-of-the-Night and Early-Morning Wakings

I like shirts with words. I've never met a shirt or sweater with "Ciao" or "Hey" or "Je t'aime" or "Mother of Dragons" that I didn't like. I love every single concert T-shirt or national park sweatshirt or Broadway musical hoodie that I own. Now that I live in California, where casual is always the style of the day, and since I have a private practice where I determine my own dress code, I even wear those T-shirts to work sometimes, though I often second-guess myself. I used to have a sweater that said "JOY" in big red capital letters, and I wore it during the winter holidays. I loved that thing until I didn't, and I've never forgotten the day it changed.

A few years after becoming a full-fledged psychologist but before I had my own kids, a psychology student was observing me on the first day of her sleep rotation. We were talking with a mom about her neurodiverse six-year-old son's sleep problems in a cramped clinic exam room, and he was becoming increasingly energetic, agitated, and loud. She described his good bedtime routine and said that he fell asleep independently. Even with good habits, he still woke several times during the night. Wanting to make the visit as short as possible to spare this poor family, I gave suggestions for sprucing up his (already good) sleep hygiene. Apparently, she'd heard this advice a hundred times already, and she'd had all she could take.

She yelled, "This is the same old thing! I've tried all this! *Nothing you are saying is going to help!* You and your 'JOY' shirt. I'm not working with anyone who wears a dumb shirt like that. I'm not talking to you. I'm only talking to her." She pointed at the student, who had no idea what to do.

I told this mom we'd be right back, and we stepped out to talk to the physician, as we usually did. I told him that she hated my "JOY" sweater. He chuckled, and after hearing about this boy's sleep, he agreed that making some small changes to sleep hygiene was a good place to start, though it was unlikely to be a magic cure. All three of us walked back into the room.

"I am not working with this girl in the 'JOY' shirt," she said, still not having it. "I'll talk with either of you but not her. I can't stand that shirt. You and your damn joy. How are you going to wear a shirt like that when you have no idea what people are going through? I'll have joy when I get some sleep."

That last part pierced me like a dart. I got it. I thought everyone would get more out of this appointment if the physician took over, and so I thanked the family, stepped out of the room, and changed my shirt in the bathroom. When the physician came out, he told me that he had pretty much said the same things I had said, and the mom was OK with it. But he added, "She really hated your 'JOY' shirt."

I can empathize with that mom because I have been annoyed with the same old suggestions, too. Henry has long struggled with not eating enough, and I feel like we have tried everything. At some especially rough points, we have seen a nutritionist, but it hasn't helped yet. I understand that putting butter on the broccoli would add calories, but then Henry wouldn't touch it. I know smoothies are a great way to sneak in protein and fat, but Henry will only drink one a few times a year. I have spent hundreds of dollars on high-calorie drink supplements that sit around until they expire, and I have added gross calorie boosters to pancakes and waffles until Henry decided they both were on his "hell no" list of foods.

Henry's developmental pediatrician gets it. When we saw her regarding his weight, she went through the usual recommendations for upping his calories, listened to me, and kept the dialogue going until we both reached the same place. That place was to give Henry unlimited quantities of the foods he likes. Granted, his favorite two foods are salmon and broccoli, but there have been glorious months when I worried less because he ate a half pound of bacon a day or a bagel with actual butter (!) for every breakfast. Because of this, I appreciate the frustration parents must feel when they hear the same tired, worn-out sleep hygiene advice. At the same time, even for neurodiverse kids, good sleep hygiene and positive sleep associations are necessary, though they may not be enough on their own. I work with many parents who have tried a million things to lessen their neurodiverse child's night wakings. They might balk at every recommendation I have, but if they are willing, I keep going until we connect somewhere, like our developmental pediatrician did with me.

Troubleshooting Night Wakings

I bet you, like the mom who hated my "JOY" sweater, don't want to hear the same sleep advice you've already heard, either. So, once your child is falling asleep at bedtime in the best possible way, if there are leftover night wakings and/or an awful early-morning wake-up time (that most people consider middle of the night), first consider why. Whenever I hear that a family has a consistent bedtime routine, their child is falling asleep completely independently, and they are still having night or early-morning wakings, I consider four possibilities:

1. They are almost there! They should keep going for another week or so to see if the child's skills generalize and naturally spill over into the rest of the night.

2. They need to directly fade their presence during those night wakings.

3. Something about the bedtime routine is sabotaging learning to self-soothe.

4. The leftover wakings are the result of having a neurodiverse brain, and we might need to think differently.

Let's start with possibility number 1: The child just needs more time and is almost at the finish line. In this situation, it might feel like working on bedtime has been happening forever, but consider how long it has been since the child has fallen asleep 100 percent on their own, starting from wide awake. If it hasn't been a full three weeks, or if there has been some interruption to the routine, stay consistent with the bedtime changes for another week or two. If it has been a full three weeks, and the skills haven't generalized to the middle of the night on their own, you are in situation number 2, and it's time to work on them directly. In this case, when your child wakes at night, gradually help them learn to return to sleep the same way they fall asleep at bedtime (see chapter 13).

Fading Night Wakings in Older Kids

For kids who come to your room when they wake, walk them back to their bed, give a quick tuck in, and shorten the time you stay each night. When you can leave right after the tuck in and they still stay in their bed, switch to walking them halfway back to their room. When they have mastered that, give them a hug from your bed, and encourage them to walk back to their room on their own and tuck themselves back in. Eventually, encourage your child to stay in their bed instead of coming to your room. If they call for you, reassure them through the monitor, or just yell loud enough so that they can hear from their bedroom — as long as it doesn't wake everyone else. A second option is to put a sleeping bag and/ or camping mattress on the floor of your bedroom. If your child wakes during the night, they don't have to wake you! They can just get in the sleeping bag and go back to sleep. Over time, you can move the sleeping bag closer and closer to their room.

When the Bedtime Routine Is the Problem

The third possibility is what I see most often: Something about the bedtime routine is sabotaging self-soothing. Because we want this process to be as easy as possible on our child, sometimes we unintentionally cheat. For instance, some people rock their child until they are nearly asleep, and then they wake them enough to open their eyes for a nanosecond, and then put them in the crib "wide awake." If your child falls asleep within seconds of being put in their bed, they are likely too drowsy to learn anything, including how to fall asleep on their own. Regardless of what other people say, my belief is that the child must learn to go from wide awake to calm to drowsy and then to fully asleep all by themselves for those sleep skills to transfer to the middle of the night.

If your child is truly falling asleep from wide awake at bedtime, consider your child's sleep associations. Paradoxically, the thing families fear stopping is usually *the* thing they need to eliminate for their child to learn to fall asleep and be able to return to sleep independently. If you think, "If we get rid of X, they'll never fall asleep," or "They fall asleep on their own except for X," then X is *the thing* to eliminate. For example, a child might fall asleep with the light from a toy aquarium or with lullabies from a stuffed caterpillar that turn off after forty-five minutes. Oops, that aquarium or caterpillar has sabotaged learning to fall asleep independently. Whether your child is being put to bed too drowsy to learn or they have an unrecognized sleep association to something they can't get for themselves at 3 a.m., they haven't learned their own self-soothing skills. To fix this, follow the advice in chapter 13.

When Night Waking Results from a Neurodiverse Brain

The fourth possibility can be the hardest: What if the wakings are the result of a neurodiverse brain? In this case, whether you are there or not, whether they have a bottle or no bottle, the iPad or no iPad, X or no X, it doesn't change their sleep pattern. They take more than forty-five minutes to fall asleep and/or get back to sleep regardless of who is there, what is happening, or what the environment is like. In this situation, a child may be awake for three hours vocalizing or looking at their hands regardless of whether a parent intervenes.

If a neurodiverse child or teen is sleeping less than we think they should be due to a late bedtime or long night wakings, we assess their daytime functioning. If shorter sleep is not leading to sleepiness or problems with mood or functioning during the day, we may shift the goal from making sure the child sleeps for ten hours in a row to making sure they are safe during long night wakings and preserving the sleep of the rest of the household. If your child wakes in the morning on their own, there is no difference in their behavior whether they have a good night of sleep or not, and they are happy and alert during the day, they may be getting the sleep they need. If it is impossible to wake your child in the morning, you notice a drastic difference in mood and/or behavior after an unusual (especially good or especially horrible) night of sleep, or they are falling asleep during the day outside of age-appropriate naps, then the amount of sleep they're getting at night is not enough.

It may be that the child takes a long time to fall asleep because bedtime is too early. They might not have enough sleep pressure yet. For example, if your child is consistently in bed by 9 p.m. but rarely falls asleep before 11:30 p.m., consider moving the bedtime routine closer to the time they are currently falling asleep. That way they are not awake in bed for long periods of time, which can lead to a negative sleep association between the bed and trouble falling asleep. If you as the parent still need child-free time from 9 to 11 p.m., perhaps put on a movie or set up another engaging solo activity for your child.

If consistent early waking is the issue, some families I've worked with have a special (but not too special) basket of toys or books or fidgets that their child can use until it's time for everyone else to start their day. Some parents switch nights or parts of the night; one sleeps with earplugs, a white noise machine, and in a different room, while the other monitors the child for safety. Other parents bring their child into their (the parents') bed, lock the door so the child is secure in the same room, and put on a show so the rest of the family can continue sleeping.

Locking doors, whether yours or your child's, is something many families wonder about, and it can be a highly charged decision. For the average child, I don't recommend locking their bedroom door for many reasons, such as the ability to get out quickly in an emergency. But for some families of neurodiverse children, there are substantial overnight safety concerns. Parents may worry that their child will leave the house or that, even with cabinets secured, they will get into dangerous items, such as cleaning supplies, sharp objects, medications, and so on. In these situations, keeping a child's door secured while also checking in with a monitor, camera, or regular visits may be the safest option. Families have to balance everyday risks with the safety issues unique to their child.

There's no right answer here, only what works best for your family's sleep and safety.

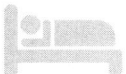

Tuck-In Tips

- Bedtime sleep skills usually generalize to the rest of the night on their own. If this hasn't happened, manage night wakings directly with the same approach you used at bedtime.

- Learning self-soothing skills can be sabotaged if your child is too drowsy or has unrecognized sleep associations.
- If your child wakes in the morning on their own and is wide awake with no change in behavior during the day, this may be their body's sleep schedule.
- Maintaining everyone's safety and maximizing sleep for the rest of the household are important considerations.

Pillow Point

Persistent night wakings can have multiple causes, including neurodivergence, and families may need to manage them in unconventional ways to maximize both sleep and safety for everyone in the house.

Chapter 15

Nighttime Fears, Worries, and Distressing Thoughts

It is 100 percent OK to comfort your child when they're afraid at night. For the very short term, this may involve a tuck in and a kiss or staying with them until they are asleep in your bed or theirs.

That said, I've seen more families than I can count where the sleep problem started with attentive parents wanting to soothe away lingering fears of that burglar or monster. The problem occurs when this soothing goes on night after night and the child develops an association between sleep and the parent. Then the child legitimately can't fall asleep without a parent being present, even if that parent prefers to sleep separately.

Kids learn quickly what to say to get what they need and want; it's adaptive. Say please and you can have a cookie. Say you're scared and a parent will sleep with you. One family I worked with years ago pulled out all the stops to manage their six-year-old's fear of the dark. Sleep had never been Sid's thing, but once he said that he was scared, the family's routines revolved around minimizing his nighttime fears. In other words, Sid now slept with his mom every night. Sid's mom was conflicted about co-sleeping. She slept best in her own bed alone, but she also felt guilty. Part of her believed that since she was a single mom and had room in her bed, she should let Sid sleep there if he wanted. Sid was an extremely restless sleeper, and his mom was a light sleeper who could not function well with less than eight solid hours of sleep per night.

Sid's dad was willing and able to have Sid sleep at his house, but he just couldn't sleep without his mom. Time after time, his parents tried to find out what exactly he was afraid of, but he couldn't really say much other than, "I'm scared." Both parents came together to address Sid's sleep fears. They gave him a plushie version of his favorite superhero, Captain America, to protect him, got a very bright nightlight for his room, used "monster spray" to keep the monsters at bay, gave him a superpower smoothie as a bedtime snack, and read stories to him about being brave at night. Nothing seemed to help. As soon as Sid was tucked in and lights were out, he would cry and yell until his mom would give in and say, "Just get into my bed."

During one impromptu family meeting, Sid told his parents that he was afraid of a googly-eyed monster he had seen on a DVD cartoon weeks prior. They asked him to draw the monster, so he did. Then the three of them made the monster silly by adding more googly eyes, yellow polka dots, a LeBron James jersey, and a grass skirt. Everyone laughed, but that night Sid still said he was scared and refused to sleep alone. The next day, Sid's parents talked about taking him to a child psychologist, but first his mom wanted to bury that googly-eyed, grass skirt–wearing monster for good. After school, Sid and his mom went to the backyard, and with a hammer, they took turns smashing the DVD to bits. Then they dug a hole deep into the ground and buried the DVD bits as well as the monster drawing so the googly eyes would never be seen again. Still, nothing changed about Sid's sleep. After talking with the family in the sleep clinic, it was clear that Sid and his mom needed to move out of that monster-infested pit immediately and buy a new house where all three of them could live together again. Obviously, I'm kidding, but that was Sid's secret hope. And while the googly-eyed monster may have started as a fear, it had become a way to delay bedtime, sleep in his mom's bed, and bring both of his parents together to deal with his nighttime fears.

The good thing about these situations is that whether a child is legitimately afraid, is trying to delay bedtime, or has a sleep association involving a parent, the way to fix it is the same: gradually increase the child's independence (and decrease parental presence) at bedtime. If they are scared, this is the way to face it, and if it is a habit or sleep association, this is the way to change it.

After a few false starts, Sid gradually learned to fall asleep at bedtime with his mom sitting in the doorway, and after several days, once she tucked him into bed, he was able to fall asleep on his own. The following week, Dad came to Mom's house at bedtime so Sid could get used to Dad putting him to bed. Once he could fall asleep 100 percent by himself, he stayed in his bed all night long. A few weeks later Sid was spending the weekdays with Mom, and every other weekend with Dad, and he could sleep on his own all night in both places. There were multiple factors that set Sid's sleep difficulties in motion, but what started with nighttime fears ended with a negative sleep association.

Nighttime Fears

Nearly three-quarters of school-age children report having nighttime fears, and often they learn to manage them on their own.[1] According to kids themselves, common helpful strategies include distraction (50 percent), talking to parents (27.9 percent), and hugging stuffed animals (9.3 percent). Even though I'm a psychologist and I encourage people to talk all day long, my advice is to avoid talking too much about the content of nighttime fears, especially at bedtime. Just like the right amount of distraction, neurodiverse kids need the right amount of reassurance to feel safe at bedtime. Counterintuitively, too much reassurance can lead to increased anxiety. Remind your child that being brave means doing something even if you are scared. Briefly assure them that they are safe, that everyone has trouble sleeping sometimes, and that you know they have the power to be brave. Then move on to a new topic. If they ask the same question repeatedly, with kindness say something like, "What did I say last time you asked me?"

Neurodiverse kids and teens can be big thinkers with big worries and even bigger feelings. If they can write or draw, have a designated book where they can jot down worries as they come up. During the day or in the evening *before* bedtime, have a special time to talk about fears and to practice ways to keep their brain calm and busy while waiting for sleep. Talk with your child about what their favorite superhero, character, or person would do if they were scared at bedtime. Have them repeat positive and true thoughts to themselves so they remember them at bedtime; something like, "I'm afraid, but I'm brave too and I can stay in my bed" or "My body feels scared, but I am safe, calm, and cozy." Older kids laugh and roll their eyes if I suggest "At bedtime, I'm a warrior, not a worrier," but I still like it.

Books about nighttime fears can also be helpful guides. Two books for elementary-aged children are *Uncle Lightfoot, Flip That Switch* by Mary F. Coffman and *What to Do When You Dread Your Bed* by Dawn Huebner.

At this point, you know I like science, so what does the research say about nighttime fears? Rarely do I think of science as cute, but studies show that stuffed animals can reduce nighttime fears. One study found that nighttime fear and anxiety were significantly reduced with a stuffed animal (the huggy puppy), whether the child was told to take care of the puppy or told that the puppy would take care of them.[2] And it doesn't have to be a plushie or a puppy. Some neurodiverse kids I've worked with prefer cars, trucks, dolls, even empty sippy cups — and as long as the objects are safe, those are great, too.

A flashlight scavenger hunt in the bedroom when it's dark (but before bedtime) is another trick for lessening nighttime fears. This should be a short activity (ten minutes or less) that you and your child do together once every day. First, hide favorite toys around the room where your child sleeps. Then use a flashlight to find the toys in the dark together. As your child gets more comfortable, have them start looking for the hidden toys alone while a parent stands in the doorway, and eventually stands in the hallway. For extra motivation, when they can be alone in the dark, hide a new toy to find.

Social Stories to Help Cope with Nighttime Fears

Social stories about coping with nighttime fears can be read with a parent, at any point in the routine before the child gets into bed. Two examples are shown below. The first is for children who might learn better with pictures or images. Both stories can be read to the child or by the child, but the stories themselves are in the first person, as if they are what the child is saying.

Story for Younger Children
I am safe and cozy in my bed at night. I might feel afraid, but I know I am OK.
My dog stuffie protects me, so I give him a big hug. My parents also keep me safe.
My parents might still be awake for a little while doing grown-up things like laundry, work, or watching a show. I can be brave and stay in my bed.

Everyone in my family sleeps at night. Even when they are sleeping, I am safe. I can wake my parents if I am sick or have an emergency.

If I wake up, I stop! I stay in my bed. I can hug my dog stuffie.

I can be brave like a superhero.

My parents will be proud of me for staying in my bed! When I wake in the morning, we will all feel rested and happy.

Story for Older Kids

- When I am in my bed at night with my puppy stuffie, I am safe. I am brave and I can do hard things.
- Sometimes my brain tricks me into thinking there are scary things in my room, but I can teach my brain that I'm safe. Even if I feel afraid of the dark, I stay in my bed. I can boss my brain back and tell it, "I am safe and cozy in my bed," or "My parents are right next door!" or "It might be dark, but I am safe and OK."
- My mom or dad might still be awake doing grown-up things like cleaning the dishes, doing laundry, or watching a grown-up show.
- Sometimes I don't feel tired. That is OK! I wait quietly with my eyes closed in my bed for sleep to come. I imagine

riding my bike or think about parts of a motorcycle while I'm waiting for sleep.

- After I fall asleep the first time, I might wake up again. I know it is not time to get up if my green light is off. I can give my dog stuffie a hug, close my eyes, and wait quietly in my bed for sleep to come again.
- I stay in my bed all night unless I feel sick or I have an emergency. I can wake Mom or Dad if I feel sick or have an emergency.
- When I see that my green light is on, it is OK to get up! When I get a good night's sleep, I feel happy and awake. The rest of my family is happy when they get a good night's sleep, too.

Worries About Sleep

Obviously, in this book, I want to emphasize how important sleep is to children and teens. But when worries about falling sleep, getting enough sleep, or being sleepy interfere with sleep itself, change the channel and avoid focusing on sleep. Encourage your child *not* to track sleep with a Fitbit or other tracking device. Discourage checking the time after lights are out. If they have a regular clock, cover it with a towel or pillowcase at bedtime and put it out of reach. Have them charge their phone and other devices in another room. Like nighttime fears, sleep worries should be discussed before bedtime. Talk about what helps your child feel awake during the day other than sleep. Sunlight, food, going outside, talking with friends, exercise, and favorite activities are examples. Talk about what makes them feel sleepy besides not getting enough sleep. Rainy days, sad thoughts, and not exercising also make us tired. Work with your child to generate one or two statements that are positive and true, such as "Even when sleep takes a long time to arrive, I'm OK," or "I'm still good at soccer, even when I'm tired."

Encourage your child to repeat these statements to themselves throughout the day, so they are easy to remember at night.

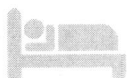

Tuck-In Tips

- Most school-age children have nighttime fears.
- Brief reassurance is helpful, but too much reassurance can increase anxiety.
- Talk with your child about nighttime worries and practice ways to handle fears *before* bedtime. Books about nighttime fears, brave talk, a flashlight scavenger hunt, and stuffed animal bodyguards can help.
- When worries are about sleep itself, minimize the focus on sleep. Avoid tracking sleep and checking the time.

Pillow Point

Nighttime fears and worries about sleep are common, and the best time to talk about them and practice coping strategies is any time before bedtime.

Chapter 16

Sensory Sensitivities and Stims

I was a modern dancer long before I was a psychologist. When I went to graduate school the first time, it was for dance. My first dance class was at age four, and my last dance performance was at age twenty-eight-ish. As I got older and started thinking about having children, in addition to imagining the homemade organic unprocessed food I would make, I also imagined the dance parties we would have. I would hear a song and get lost thinking about dancing with my yet-unborn child. When Henry was just a baby, I noticed he was attuned to music, and I took him to a baby music class. When I told the teacher about how Henry responded to music, and that I thought he might have a natural affinity for it, she was unimpressed. She vaguely nodded and said that all babies like music. Henry loved listening to kid music at home, which we did pretty much all day every day. In line with my dreams, I danced all over the house with him.

A year or two later, as I was trying to figure out what was going on with Henry's development, we were still taking music class with the same teacher. We had been going consistently and had met our best family friends there. On this particular day, the teacher dumped out a box of kid-friendly instruments like maracas, tambourines, triangles, and so on, and all the other kids started experimenting with making sounds. Henry, on the other hand, organized the instruments into piles based on whether they had any features that looked like eyes. Uh-oh, I thought.

The next year, after we were well into our routine of therapies, Henry still loved music, and we thought he might like music lessons. The teacher, Abhi, was fantastic, and the exercises he taught Henry on the piano were easy and fun. Henry had specific ideas about what he wanted his music lesson to be, and this included the guitar, which thankfully the teacher played. Henry wanted Abhi to play the entire Beatles catalog on the guitar and sing, while he memorized the lyrics from the pages in front of him. We started with "Yellow Submarine" and worked our way through "Octopus's Garden" and even "Norwegian Wood." I was singing Beatles songs day and night. Those were the days.

Soon after the days of the Beatles, Henry became extremely sensitive to sounds, and any music became unbearable for him. We took him to a live concert of the kids' band the Okee Dokee Brothers, which was his favorite kids' band prior to the Beatles. He previously loved seeing the Okee Dokee Brothers live, but now he couldn't tolerate it for even five minutes, and we had to leave. For the next many years, to avoid meltdowns, we avoided music, even the radio.

Then when Henry was in fourth grade, his school offered an orchestra class and music lessons, and Henry wanted to participate. I looked at the list of possible instruments and uploaded videos of people playing each one. I showed him, and when we got to the cello, he excitedly said, "That's the one! That's it! I love the cello!" I was happy that he had made his way back to music. I immediately pushed my luck by playing "Like a Prayer" in the kitchen. I danced around, taking his hands in mine and encouraging him to dance with me, but he ran away. Maybe no dancing, I thought, but at least he wanted to try a musical instrument. I was all-in with this cello business and even found a cello teacher to give lessons at home to help him with his school orchestra songs. The only way this teacher could get Henry to even attempt to play the school songs was to first teach him snippets of songs he loved. So I would hear sounds from the online game *Among Us* and the cello version of Snoop

Dogg's "What's My Name?," and then I would hear groaning and eventually "Mary Had a Little Lamb."

One October day, Henry's class was learning holiday songs for the winter chorus concert, and apparently Henry disrupted the class by sobbing and yelling, "It's not even Halloween yet!" He couldn't calm down, and I was called to bring my sweet kid home from school because he was so upset. In my mind, I thought, *Well, at least we have the cello*, which obviously jinxed it. Soon after, we got a note from the orchestra teacher telling us Henry wasn't playing his instrument during class, and she encouraged us to withdraw him from orchestra. I asked if he was disrupting the class or bothering anyone, and she said, "No, he just sits there." Um, OK. What's the problem? Throw us a bone here! I declined and kept him in the class until a few months later when he was officially kicked out of orchestra for not playing.

I talked to him about it, reminding him that he picked the cello. "You told me you loved the sound of it, remember?" I showed him the video we had watched together months before, and he clarified, "What I meant was that I like the sound of the word *cello*, not the sound of the cello."

Oh. If he had a mic, it would have dropped right there.

Families with a Neurodiverse Child

I was once reading a study about how the sensory sensitivities of neurodiverse kids impact the whole family,[1] and I thought, *That's us!* Three main themes emerged from what the families described, which I doubt will be surprising. First, the families decided what activities to do together based on how much sensory overload there might be and their estimate of whether their neurodiverse child could cope. Second, neurotypical family members felt sad about not being able to share meaningful events, emotions, memories, and conversations as a whole family. This was either because their neurodiverse sibling or child couldn't participate or because a parent had to be focused on the neurodiverse child and couldn't participate. For example, eating together in restaurants, attending sporting events, and being together at family reunions or weddings are situations that are often difficult for neurodiverse kids and their families. Last, the families in the study planned activities in advance — making sure they had earplugs, headphones, dry clothes, snacks from home, sunglasses, hats, extra jackets, and that one special water bottle.

The need for preparation strongly resonates with me. I remember an especially happy excursion for our family, a monster truck rally. Both of my kids have loved playing with monster trucks since they were itty-bitty. When I saw that their favorites — Grave Digger, El Toro Loco, and Higher Education — were going to be at a stadium near us, I immediately bought tickets. I got excited the way I still do when I pass a construction site, before I realize I no longer have toddlers in the back seat to appreciate the backhoe and dump trucks. I was jazzed for about two minutes until it hit me that this event was going to be loud, *really* loud. I started preparing immediately by ordering five different kinds of earplugs and headphones. When they arrived, we tested them to see if Henry would be able to wear the noise-canceling earbuds with headphones on top for extra soundproofing. We paid in advance for preferred parking in case we had to leave early. Our seats were near the quiet room of the stadium (it was a very forward-thinking stadium), which was amazing.

Finally, the day came and we were all excited. We drove an hour to the stadium, walked to the door, and then I realized I left the bag with all the supplies at home. We had no noise-canceling earbuds, no headphones, no snacks, and no extra sweatshirt. All I had were my purple foam earplugs in the pocket of my new hoodie, which I now planned to give Henry to wear if he needed it. We got to our seats, I shoved down my expectations and my nerves, and then I accidentally dropped my brand-new hoodie into the large puddle of beer in front of my seat. It was now too wet and stinky for Henry. This day was becoming a complete and total mom fail, until it became an *awesome* surprise. I put my foam earplugs in Henry's ears. We sat down, and I feel like the next sentence should be in a different color, with huge font, bold, underlined, and italicized: I did not hear one single word of complaining for three hours! Not from any member of our family. The monster trucks were so riveting that they eclipsed Henry's sensory overload.

Contrary to the saying, I didn't prepare for the worst, but I still hoped for the best, and it happened!

Sensory Sensitivities and Sleep

Strong sensory sensitivities and preferences are often part of neurodiversity, and sleep routines are laden with sensory experiences that tend to either promote or interfere with sleep. These sensory preferences are sometimes put into categories as "sensory seeking" or "sensory avoiding," but in my work and in my parenting, I just think of them in terms of whether they help or don't help sleep. Science has shown us that sensory sensitivities and sleep problems go together for neurodiverse people from infancy through adulthood.[2] When sensory sensitivities improve, sleep improves, and when sensory sensitivities worsen, sleep worsens. Knowing this, how can we manage the sensory aspects of the bedtime routine and the sleep environment so that our neurodiverse child or teen can get the best sleep? In chapter 11, I describe the ideal sleep environment as quiet, dark, cool, and comfortable.[3] For neurodiverse kids, it might help to keep the bedroom walls empty so there isn't anything cool or entertaining to look at, and to avoid having books or toys in the room.

Neurodiverse people can be extra sensitive to sound, and this can absolutely get in the way of sleep. Though our brains are supposed to turn sound down during sleep, this doesn't always happen for people with neurodevelopmental conditions. Also, houses and neighborhoods can be noisy! Studies of sleep in the general population of children show that noise in the neighborhood from people, emergency vehicles, cars, or airplanes can interfere with sleep.[4] One way to manage this is with continuous sound, such as from a sound machine or a fan.[5] Put these devices somewhere central in the room to mask the noises inside your house and outside in the neighborhood. Make sure that whatever sound you choose stays the same all night, which is why an audiobook or playlist is not ideal. Remember that whatever is present at bedtime is what is needed to quickly get back to sleep during normal night wakings. Otherwise, keep the volume moderate and use whatever sound or fan you like. There are also noise-canceling headphones and earbuds, even for side sleepers, that might help to keep out sounds that interfere with sleep; however, these haven't been studied in pediatrics.

When it comes to touch, research shows that massage, especially Qigong and Thai massage before bed, can have a positive impact on the sleep of children with ADHD, ASD, and other developmental delays.[6] While you could use that as an excuse to go to Thailand to study massage, research has shown that parents can be trained in about three hours, and that incorporating a fifteen-minute massage into the bedtime routine most nights led to improvements in the child's sleep. In my office, families have reported good experiences with deep pressure, such as rolling their child into a blanket like a burrito and snuggling them or doing joint compressions. Other families have told me that a few minutes on a lateral swing, play time with kinetic sand or Play-Doh, or watching videos of fish in the ocean helped their neurodiverse children calm down prior to bedtime.

People ask about weighted blankets and vests a lot, and the research is mixed.[7] The vests should not be worn during sleep for safety reasons, but there is a smidge of evidence demonstrating they may help when worn before bed. There is more evidence to suggest that weighted blankets might help sleep but not enough for me to firmly recommend a weighted blanket, and they are expensive! I recommend asking your child's occupational therapist or other trusted team member about it, and if you can, borrow one to try it out.

I often suggest a sensory calm-down routine, not only to help with sleep but just because most people enjoy it. This routine might include smelling a candle, essential oil, or slice of citrus; petting the dog; or touching a sequin pillow or fuzzy sweater. Have your child or teen pick the scent of their soap or the flavor of their toothpaste. Create a sensory calm-down box to play with before bedtime, including different textured fabrics, squishy balls or animals, a silky ribbon or tag, a soft-colored light, and a bell or chime. If your child is soothed by touching Velcro strips or sensory strips, consider putting some on the wall or bed that they can touch at night. According to neurodiverse teens (you'll hear more about this in chapter 20), other ways to find sensory engagement before bed include: cold fruit or popsicles for bedtime snack, pj's with big satin tags, pj's without any tags, holding a stuffed animal or pillow, smelling something good, tracing the edges of the bed with fingers or just with eyes, and using a sound machine.[8]

Stims or Self-Stimulating Behaviors

Repetitive self-stimulating behaviors, or stims, are a core symptom of ASD and are also common (though usually not as public) in people with ADHD. These stims help people with ASD and ADHD regulate emotions, deal with sensory overload, reduce anxiety, and increase focus.[9] Many of the neurodivergent adolescents and young adults I've worked with have shared that they get a burst of excitement or energy when they get into bed, and they handle it by rocking, rubbing their legs, rolling back and forth, snapping, humming, or any other stim. They can't sleep until they do a certain amount of stimming, even if they try to stop. I'm in the camp that believes we shouldn't try to stop stims, but we can try to replace them if the stim is waking others or is self-injurious, which is serious. Ideas that have worked for my family include having one or more fidgets in bed, having a textured squeeze ball to roll on, or writing the alphabet with fingers on the palm or arm of the other hand.

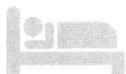

Tuck-In Tips

- One person's sensory sensitivities impact the whole family.
- Sensory sensitivities and sleep problems tend to go together. Address sensory elements that worsen your child's sleep such as traffic noise, scratchy blankets, or seamed socks.
- Sensory engagement can help prepare neurodiverse people for sleep, but what works is specific to each individual.
- Stims may help with falling asleep and are difficult to stop.

Pillow Point

Add sensory components to the bedtime routine and address sensory sensitivities that impact sleep, especially noise.

Chapter 17

Movement and Mindfulness

I love yoga and mindfulness meditation, and I feel much better physically, mentally, and emotionally when I regularly practice both. When my children were in preschool and first grade, I fantasized about how great family yoga could be at the beginning of our bedtime routine, all of us calming down together, focusing on our breath, and doing a few relaxing poses. After that, the kids would drift easily off to a peaceful slumber, and I would eat chocolate and read my book in bed alone (ha ha). For real, I did investigate what yoga poses might help sleep and how to adapt them for kids. I made a handout to give to families at work and to show my own kids our new yoga routine.

The first night we tried this, my kids were extra energetic and silly even before starting, but I decided to go for it anyway. We started with our sun breath, reaching to the sky, and then starfish, extending all five points. We stood strong in mountain pose and held each other's hands while we lifted one leg and then the other like birds. We moved smoothly through the poses, and by the time we got to child's pose, both of my kids asked to go to bed! *Not.*

What happened was that at the first mention of breath, they started snorting like pigs, trying to get boogies on each other and laughing. During starfish, their goal was to poke each other in the ribs without moving their feet. They refused to hold hands during bird and tree and instead tried to yank each other off balance. Wow, did the wheels come off during ladybug, with hysterical laughter leading to a pee accident. I decided to abandon bedtime yoga that night, but after everyone was cleaned up and dressed, my little yogis were running around buzzing like bees and stinging me. They were too busy meowing and mooing to do the cat/cow pose, and I would have needed a tranquilizer to get them calm enough for child's pose. Years later, what strikes me is not that bedtime yoga helped sleep (it didn't), but how wonderful it was that my kids played *with* each other and cooperated in their silliness. Their interaction has always been sparse but seems especially rare lately, and I find myself thinking about trying a regular yoga practice with them again for a different purpose.

Though my first experience with bedtime yoga wasn't successful, legitimate research reinforces that yoga helps neurodiverse kids with executive functioning, repetitive behaviors, social skills, and...sleep. In one study, yoga twice a week at school improved nighttime sleep in school-age children with ASD and/or ADHD.[1] The Get Ready Project (www.thegetreadyproject.com) started as a thirty-minute daily yoga program for preschoolers with ASD, and it has grown to include all neurodiverse kids.[2] They offer five- to ten-minute yoga "ready break" videos for different times of day on their website. There are countless other videos, books, blogs, and TikTok videos with ideas for yoga and sleep. Though no one method stands out, a combination of easy stretching poses and focused breathing can bring on the calm before sleep. Needless to say, I would recommend experimenting with bedtime yoga poses during the day first, so that you can identify the most calming poses for your child and leave out the ones that lead to chaos.

In addition to yoga, all types of exercise — including biking, running, and swimming — have clear, broad benefits on motor skills, coordination, social skills, behavioral problems, and sleep in neurodiverse kids, teens, and adults.[3] Jogging thirty minutes a day for twelve weeks has been shown to increase melatonin and total sleep time in kids with ASD.[4] What neurodiverse kids do during the day impacts how they sleep at night, and unquestionably, exercise helps them sleep.

Mindfulness

You might think that mindfulness is a lofty state for any child to attempt, let alone a neurodiverse child. A few studies demonstrate that, not only can children with ADHD and ASD learn mindfulness techniques, but these techniques help kids stay off the emotional teeter-totter by regulating emotions, decreasing aggressive behavior, and improving sleep.[5] Mindfulness is about internal awareness, and so it's valuable to know what parents and kids think about it. After teaching mindfulness for several weeks, one study asked parents and their neurodiverse kids if and how it was helpful. While of course the answers were all over the place, many of the themes related to relaxation: pausing, getting back to the present, acceptance, deciding what to do next, feeling calm, and responding calmly.[6] When I work with impulsive kids, we try to find that tiny space between the triggering event or feeling and the blowup. Skills like controlled breathing and increasing awareness can help to keep the spark small, before it becomes a raging fire. Introduce mindfulness skills during the day, and then bring them to bedtime, which can be full of sparks. Since defining mindfulness can be tricky, I like to talk about the concrete elements that can help sleep: breathing, awareness, and connection.

Breathing Techniques

How you practice breathing techniques with your child depends on their age, what they can do, what they like, and how long they can tolerate it. One option is to sit near your child while they're doing something else and breathe slowly and calmly. You might use a prop such as a Hoberman sphere (expanding and contracting the flexible toy as you breath in and out) and/or narrate what you're doing. The wonderful book *Alphabreaths* by my friend Dr. Chris Willard illustrates a different type of breathing for each letter of the alphabet. I pretty much learned everything I know about using mindfulness with children from Chris, and I have found all his books to be helpful.

Many different breathing techniques use the same common pattern: inhale slowly, pause, and exhale even more slowly. Here are several variations. Practice each one for a minute or for as long as you and your child can tolerate it. The duration of the practice depends on your child's age and attention.

> **Box breathing:** This method alternates inhales and exhales with pauses of equal lengths (like four sides of a box). Inhale to a count of four, pause for four, exhale for four, and pause for four, then repeat the sequence.
>
> **7-4-7:** Inhale for a count of seven, hold for four, and exhale for seven. I pick the numbers with the child or teen, so it's at their pace.
>
> **Stuffie breathing:** Lie down and put a stuffed animal on your belly. As you breathe in, watch it go up, and as you breath out, watch it go down.
>
> **Color breathing:** What's your favorite calm color? As you breathe in, imagine the color spreading calm throughout your body. As you exhale, breathe out your stress.
>
> **Silent sigh:** This is a good one for school because it can be done incognito. Lace your hands together behind your head, gently press your elbows back to open your chest, and take a slow deep breath in, hold it, and slowly breathe out.
>
> **Word breath:** Pick a short word and a longer word or phrase. Breathe in the short word slowly, pause, and

then exhale the long word. One boy I worked with picked "passenger train" for the inhale and "blue and orange Chessie Systems engine" for the exhale.

Present-Moment Awareness

Multiple astute people have said that our senses are our portal to the present. I'm not sure who was first. Aristotle? Jon Kabat-Zinn? I first heard it from another student in a virtual meditation class. Especially for kids who either have a hard time moving on from something or are worried about something coming up, I like to bring them back to the present using their senses.

Here are four examples:

Feet: Notice your feet. How do they feel in your socks? Are they on the ground? If you're in bed, how do your feet feel on your sheets? What else do you notice?

What do you hear?: Start with the big picture. What does the world sound like? Then listen for closer, smaller sounds. If you get distracted, think to yourself gently: *There's the distraction again. It's OK. I can get back to listening.*

Thought watching: Notice and name your thoughts as if you were watching from outside: "I'm imagining eating pretzels," "I'm nervous about sleeping," and so on.

Progressive muscle relaxation: Start by squeezing your toes for a few seconds and then relax them. Repeat with your feet, calves, thighs, and so on. Keep going until you get to the top of your head. Then tense and relax your whole body at once. The squeezing helps us identify the muscle so that we can relax it.

Connection to Others

When bedtime is one of the most difficult times of the day, it's not an obvious time for connection. But if you can, join your child or teen in their world for a bit around bedtime. Not because it is going to transform sleep, just because. Having a parent say the same words or do the same gesture (like a hug or pat) right before bed is also helpful for sleep.[7] I love the idea of a secret sign to connect with your child at any time of day. I squeeze both my sons' hands three times, which for us means "I love you." Now when I do it, Simon rolls his eyes and says with a sigh, "I know, Mom. I love you, too." For younger school-aged children, the book *The Kissing Hand* by Audrey Penn is great, and you can incorporate any secret sign at bedtime.

There is a Buddhist meditation practice called Tonglen in which we imagine connecting our suffering to the suffering of others in order to foster compassion. I first learned about it in Pema Chödrön's book *Comfortable with Uncertainty*. It's a practice of breathing in discomfort, pain, and distress and breathing out peace and healing. I think about this practice a lot when I'm working with people with sleep problems. The idea of connecting with others in the world experiencing the same thing seems to be reassuring, even to kids. I first tried it with a few neurodiverse adolescents as just another way to slow down thoughts and calm down at bedtime and while waiting for sleep. I've kept it going because there was such a positive response despite no real scientific research.

Here's the basic script I use with adolescents:

Picture in your mind, someone that you know (it can also be an anonymous someone) who has trouble sleeping just like you. They could be feeling tired but not able to fall asleep easily, irritated about the difficulty of shutting off racing thoughts, or stressed about staying awake during class. As you are breathing in and out, imagine that your warm inhale contains that person's frustration about their sleep. Breathe it in. On the exhale, imagine you are soothing that person's distress with your long, slow, cool, healing breath. Do this a few times. Then allow yourself to connect with the stress you feel about your own challenging sleep. Breathe in the heat of it and exhale out long, slow, cool, healing breaths. Do this a few more times. Then imagine all others suffering with similar sleep challenges. There are people everywhere in the world at this very moment experiencing what you are going through. The very same sleep struggles. Take a warm, slow, deep inhale, acknowledging the frustration of people everywhere who are experiencing sleep problems, and on the exhale, breathe out your wish to ease the tension and discomfort. Continue this for several breaths, joining others just like you by inhaling the heat of the problem and breathing out the frustration and stress, imagining it evaporating into nothing. When you are finished, you can put a hand on your heart and bring your awareness back to the present.

In my experience, acknowledging that other people in the world are experiencing exactly the same sleep problems can be reassuring, especially to adolescents.

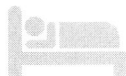

Tuck-In Tips

- Exercise of any type has been shown to improve sleep in all people, including neurodiverse kids.
- There is evidence that mindfulness techniques focusing on breath, awareness, and connection can improve sleep in neurodiverse kids.

Pillow Point

For better sleep, encourage your child to move their body as much as possible during the day, and also introduce any mindfulness techniques that are helpful for them.

Chapter 18

Melatonin, Magnesium, Marijuana, and Medications

Henry slept independently starting at seven months old, and the timing of bedtime, wake time, and naps was very consistent for at least two years. Then his sleep changed. He started waking for the day at 3 or 4 a.m., a time most people consider nighttime, and/or waking during the night for several hours. He stopped napping, which was normal for a three- to five-year-old, but he didn't sleep longer or take a nap even on days following especially rough nights. I started noticing that any challenging sensory experiences or things that were new, different, or exciting would lead to especially bad sleep, which lasted about a week. The dilemmas popped up all over the place. Do I give him the new Hot Wheels toy I bought as an incentive for peeing in the potty? Will he be awake at 3 a.m. talking and thinking about the new car for the next week? Do we let him watch the episode of *Daniel Tiger's Neighborhood* about potty training? That might be a good way to convey that even if you are playing and having fun, when you gotta go, you gotta go. Or would it lead to two to three hours of singing a new jingle in the middle of the night for days on end?

I remember the exact moment I gave in to the idea of giving Henry medications for sleep. I was walking down the hall at work with two close friends, talking about the prescribing practices of our sleep physician colleagues, especially for those families with a neurodiverse child. I thought they should be more flexible about recommending supplements and medications for certain children. Then I started complaining about being tired, and I explained Henry's tough sleep patterns. Believe it or not, I didn't consciously make the connection to what we had been discussing when I told them that I felt like it was harder for me to think lately, almost like my brain was underwater. My friends had both noticed. I explained that Henry had been waking for the day at 3 or 4 a.m. for many months, and it was taking a toll on both of us. My friend turned to me and asked, "Do you think it's time for a prescription?" I know this sounds ridiculous, but I was shocked. I responded, "I'm a behavioral sleep person. Am I really going to medicate my child?" They both chimed in at the same time, "YES!" After a lot of hemming and hawing, what ifs, and asking questions I already knew the answers to, one of them asked me what I would recommend to a patient or family in my situation. Without hesitation, I replied that if the family had exhausted (ha ha) all possibilities and had the best possible sleep habits, I would unquestionably recommend discussing melatonin and/or medications with their pediatrician.

After thinking about it for a few more months, I talked about medications with Henry's awesome developmental pediatrician, Dr. Ali Downes. She was one of the people on "team Henry" I really trusted. She recommended starting with melatonin and trying another medication if that didn't help. I had two main concerns about this plan. I wanted to make sure we weren't medicating Henry just so that *I* could get better sleep. I wanted the medication to be solely for Henry's benefit. I also wanted to make sure she wasn't prescribing a medication because I wanted her to. She nodded her head and said, "Yeah, a lot of families feel that way, but that's really not how it works."

In my practice, I've noticed that many parents are wary of discussing medications for their neurodiverse child because they worry it's for their own benefit. However, Dr. Downes was right:

That's not really how it works. There are zero providers I've encountered in my professional capacity or in my personal life who prescribe sleep medications to a child because the parents are tired. They do it to help the child.

Research has shown that most parents want to avoid giving sleep supplements or medications to their neurodiverse children.[1] Unusual reactions, side effects, and interactions with other medications can be challenging to manage, and let's face it, there is no magic potion for sleep. In the general population of US children, about one-third take a vitamin or supplement, and most of the time it is not prescribed by a medical professional.[2] My advice is to always talk to your child's medical provider about using supplements or medications, and avoid trying them as a first option. Instead, first try a behavioral approach (which is the focus of chapters 10 through 17), and have your child evaluated by their pediatrician for medical problems and sleep disorders. At that point, if your neurodiverse child still takes hours to fall asleep and/or has long night wakings or wakes too early, explore other avenues.

Before you read this chapter, I want to be crystal clear: I am not a physician, and I am not authorized or qualified to give advice about medications. My goal is to describe what's available, so you know what the options are and you can discuss them with your child's medical provider. I've provided tables throughout the book that you can take a picture of on your phone and bring with you.

Supplements

In the United States, unlike in some European countries, Canada, and Japan, supplements such as melatonin, magnesium, and other vitamins are not regulated the way over-the-counter and prescription medications are by the Food and Drug Administration (FDA).[3] Many supplements sold in the US are manufactured in China, which also does not have strict regulatory procedures.

This means that we don't know what specific brands or preparations of a given supplement are the safest or the most effective. We can't be 100 percent confident that 2 mg of a certain vitamin really contains 2 mg of that vitamin. It could be more, it could be less. This is true about multivitamins, probiotics, omega-3 supplements, and any other supplement sold in the US. We also don't know what else might be in that supplement. Even different bottles of the exact same brand, dose, and preparation can vary. For example, at least two scientific studies have shown that the gummy versions of melatonin are particularly unreliable in terms of their content.[4] In the most recent study, only three out of twenty-five tested melatonin brands had a melatonin level within 10 percent of what the label on the bottle indicated.

Studies also show that supplements often contain additional unlisted ingredients. Though the FDA requests that manufacturers list all ingredients, I'm not sure who (if anyone) is checking. Supplement studies conducted by independent organizations (not supplement companies) have found small amounts of diphenhydramine (Benadryl), arsenic, stimulants, heavy metals, and other ingredients in various supplements. Does that mean we should stay away from vitamins and supplements? I personally don't think so, but I also check to see where my vitamins are manufactured.

As you mull over what might help your child's sleep, it's important to remember that there is a lot of misinformation, even from well-meaning people. I look to the science, and I try to find studies on particular vitamins or supplements that include neurodiverse kids or teens. If there aren't any studies, that doesn't mean that supplement won't help; but it means we don't have scientific evidence that it does. Since I am not a medical provider or a supplement expert, I have to do my own research like any parent.

There are at least three independent organizations that certify that a supplement has the ingredients it claims to have, meets limits for additional ingredients and contaminants, and/or meets standards for good manufacturing practices. Those are Consumer

Lab (www.consumerlab.com), NSF International (previously called National Sanitation Foundation; www.nsf.org), and United States Pharmacopeia (USP; www.usp.org). These organizations each set their own standards, and you may want to investigate further before putting trust in their seals of approval.

Melatonin

The big supplement for sleep is melatonin. In addition to research showing the benefits of melatonin for jet lag (or acclimating to different time zones), there is a significant body of research investigating the use of melatonin to improve sleep in neurodiverse children and adolescents.[5] There is regular/immediate-release melatonin that comes in various forms, including liquid, chewable, dissolvable, capsules, and tablets. There is also continuous or extended-release melatonin; as of this writing, this only comes in a coated tablet. The coating on the tablet is what allows the melatonin to be released over time, and so it cannot be crushed. Also, regardless of what the label says, there is no special melatonin for kids. Melatonin is all the same.

The benefits of immediate-release (regular) melatonin — of 1 mg to 10 mg, administered within a few hours of bedtime — are mostly related to falling asleep, not necessarily to staying asleep. In children and adolescents with ADHD, melatonin has been shown to be effective at reducing the time it takes to fall asleep,[6] and for those who have used melatonin continuously for more than 3.5 years, it remains effective with minimal side effects.[7] Melatonin (both extended release and regular release) has been widely studied in the US, Canada, and Europe in children, teens, and adults with ADHD, ASD, Down syndrome, Smith-Magenis syndrome, Angelman syndrome, Rett syndrome, tuberous sclerosis, and Williams syndrome, to name a few. Improvements in sleep without serious side effects have been found even after two years of using extended-release melatonin in children with ASD and/or ADHD. No impact on puberty has been found in human studies, which is a concern sometimes expressed by parents.[8] Extended-release preparations of melatonin may help to reduce night wakings while the person is taking it, but once it is stopped, sleep problems tend to recur (though sleep is often better than prior to starting melatonin in the first place).

There have not been any studies reporting overdose or other serious side effects of melatonin, and there are few reports of drug interactions with melatonin.[9] According to a report by the Agency for Healthcare Research and Quality (AHRQ; a US government agency), the most commonly reported adverse effects of melatonin were nausea (1.5 percent), headache (7.8 percent), dizziness (4 percent), and drowsiness (20 percent). However, these rates were not any higher than in people given a placebo.[10] This result did not change by dose, the presence or absence of a sleep disorder, type of sleep disorder, duration of treatment, gender, age, formulation of melatonin, or use of concurrent medications.

Similarly, in children with ASD and/or ADHD, after two years of taking extended-release melatonin, no short- or long-term adverse events were reported.[11] The most common side effects were fatigue (6.3 percent), sleepiness (6.3 percent), and mood swings (4.2 percent), but again, these side effects were similar in the group that got the placebo. Other studies have found fatigue, sleepiness, mood swings, nightmares, dizziness, and earlier morning wakings.[12] In my professional experience, families have occasionally reported that melatonin seemed to increase vivid and/or weird dreams. In addition to its effects on sleep, melatonin is an antioxidant that has been shown to protect the brain from oxidative stress and inflammation in both neurodivergent and non-neurodivergent people.[13]

There are ten questions about melatonin that I'm asked most frequently, and I answer them in this handy-dandy chart:

Table 18.1: Q&A About Melatonin

Does taking melatonin...	What the science says
Stop your body from producing its own melatonin?	No, multiple long-term (up to 4.5 years) studies of continuous use melatonin have not shown this, nor have they shown that a dose increase is needed over time to sustain the same effect.
Cause nightmares?	Maybe. Nightmares and vivid dreams are primarily seen in adults but have also been reported in children.
Cause parasomnias like sleep terrors and sleep talking?	Possibly, but melatonin has also been shown to reduce parasomnias. Go figure.
Make a person feel sleepy in the morning?	Fatigue and sleepiness can be side effects. These effects tend to lessen or vanish when the dose is reduced and/or the melatonin is given earlier in the night.
Lead to addiction to melatonin supplements or other substances?	No, melatonin is not addictive, and research with adults suggests that melatonin might even be helpful in treating addiction and withdrawal.[14]
Help infants and toddlers?	Melatonin is approved in Europe for sleep problems in children age two years and above with certain neurodevelopmental conditions. It has been used for other indications in newborns and infants three months old and older without side effects.[15]
Impact puberty?	Melatonin has not been shown to impact puberty in children and teens.

Table 18.1: Q&A About Melatonin (*continued*)

Does taking melatonin...	What the science says
Worsen sleep?	Unlikely. If sleep gets worse, it's likely because a child is resistant to feeling sleepy or woozy, *or* there are other ingredients in that bottle of melatonin causing worse sleep.
Cause problems in the long run?	Melatonin has been studied for about 4.5 years of continuous use without side effects or effects on growth or puberty. Beyond that, we don't know.
Cross the blood-brain barrier?	Yes, melatonin does cross the blood-brain barrier.

There are drawbacks to melatonin supplements beyond the uncertainty around what is in a melatonin capsule, tablet, or chewable. There isn't standard dosing or timing for melatonin.[16] Studies range from using 0.5 mg to 10 mg. At higher doses, there are not necessarily more side effects, but the impact on sleep doesn't get any greater, either. Some medical professionals recommend giving melatonin three to four hours before bedtime, but most advise to give it twenty to sixty minutes before bedtime. Lacking clear guidance, it is up to parents (in consultation with medical providers) to figure out the best melatonin dose and timing for their child. Another concern about melatonin is that increasing numbers of people are taking it, and with increased use comes the inevitable increase in accidental ingestions and intentional overdoses. Melatonin overdose has not been linked to death; however, melatonin overdoses have not been widely reported and thus are not well studied.

Iron/Serum Ferritin

Numerous articles refer to mineral and vitamin deficiencies that are common in neurodiverse children, which makes sense due to picky eating from sensory sensitivities, medications, and so on. Many of these articles claim that the deficiencies cause sleep problems and that using vitamin or mineral supplements leads to improvements in sleep. Only iron has been widely studied in neurodiverse children and found to relate to sleep. Ferritin in the blood is a measure of iron storage in the body. Serum ferritin levels under 50 ng/mL are common in children with neurodevelopmental conditions and can be related to restless sleep, especially in children with ADHD (see chapter 5).[17]

A pediatrician might routinely check a child's hemoglobin/ iron levels, but ferritin is not typically ordered unless it is specifically requested. When a baby gets that heel stick to check for low iron, it doesn't tell diddly squat about ferritin. That said, I recommend consulting with a sleep provider before you request a ferritin level for your child. Why not just ask your pediatrician to order it, like I did? It makes sense to consult a sleep provider first for five reasons:

1. A ferritin level is a blood test, and no one wants to put their child through an unnecessary stick.
2. There are side effects from taking iron that neurodiverse kids are often already struggling with, like constipation.
3. It's possible to have too much iron, which can be harmful.
4. Iron supplements for sleep are different than for run-of-the-mill low iron. A sleep provider will be able to give guidelines about when, how much, what time, and what type of iron should be taken.
5. If your child does not have restless sleep, there is no solid reason to check a child's ferritin level. Many kids likely

have serum ferritin levels under 50 ng/mL, but if they don't have sleep problems, there is no need to test them.

Working in the sleep field and being curious, I asked my pediatrician to add a ferritin level for Henry as part of a routine blood test when he was a baby. Henry wasn't getting an extra stick or giving more blood, so I thought, why not? The result came back as 19 ng/mL. Since Henry wasn't having any sleep problems at that point, my pediatrician recommended doing nothing, and that's exactly what I did.

Vitamin D

There is very little research on vitamin D supplements and sleep in neurodiverse children, but in a general sample of kids, vitamin D deficiency has been associated with slightly shorter total sleep time and lower sleep efficiency (time asleep when in bed).[18] This deficiency may impact the circadian system, as a delayed bedtime has been found in children who are vitamin D deficient.[19] Children with obstructive sleep apnea, especially if they are obese, are at risk of vitamin D deficiency, and this has been linked to possible increased inflammation and more severe obstructive sleep apnea.[20]

Magnesium

I can see why magnesium seems to be everyone's new favorite supplement. The magnesium produced by our bodies does great things, such as fostering muscle relaxation, calming the nervous system, promoting muscle and nerve functioning, increasing bone strength, and maintaining healthy functioning of the heart, blood pressure, and blood sugar. In children, magnesium in combination with other medications can treat acute asthma flares and is given to mothers in preterm labor to improve brain development in preterm babies.

What does magnesium do for sleep in neurodiverse kids and teens? It's hard to know. Unlike melatonin, there isn't yet a strong foundation of research. Results of several studies have been combined and analyzed to show that children with ADHD have lower levels of magnesium compared with controls; however, the study methods were so different from each other that the authors recommend more research before drawing any conclusions.[21]

In terms of treatment, there has been at least one randomized, double-blind, placebo-controlled trial (the most stringent type of study) of magnesium and vitamin D supplementation in six-to-twelve-year-olds diagnosed with ADHD.[22] After eight weeks of treatment, magnesium and vitamin D levels were increased, and some symptoms of ADHD were decreased, including emotional and peer problems, overall problems, and internalizing problems. Treatment did not significantly impact hyperactivity, conduct problems, prosocial behaviors, or externalizing. Unfortunately, sleep was not studied. Of note, one study in adults with restless legs syndrome showed that taking a combination magnesium-citrate-and-B6 supplement helped to improve sleep quality and decrease symptoms after about two months of use.[23]

In addition to oral supplements, it has been hypothesized that a person can absorb magnesium through the skin. That means a warm bath with Epsom salts (aka magnesium sulfate), magnesium flakes, or a magnesium foot spray might be a way to increase magnesium in the body.[24] I like the idea, but it's a stretch, and there just isn't enough science for me to get on board with using magnesium to improve kids' sleep yet. On the other hand, a warm bath with Epsom salts or a gentle foot rub using a soothingly scented magnesium oil could make for a relaxing bedtime ritual — and while it may only lead to softer skin, it's unlikely to do any harm.

5-HTP/Tryptophan

There is a lot of chatter, especially around Thanksgiving, about turkey and sleepiness due to the naturally occurring tryptophan in those birds, but science doesn't tell us much about tryptophan supplements, sleep, and kids. Two supplements, 5-HTP (5-hydroxytryptophan) and L-tryptophan (both serotonin precursors), claim to improve the sleep of kids and teens, though the evidence isn't there yet. However, a smidge of science shows that a 5-HTP supplement may be effective at reducing NREM parasomnias in children, specifically sleep terrors.[25] Additionally, 5-HTP/tryptophan might impact the circadian rhythm and/or slow wave sleep. While most of the circadian research is in elderly populations, one study in children found that more than ten minutes of morning light plus a tryptophan supplement at breakfast might encourage an "early-bird" rhythm.[26] It is also likely that the light exposure itself contributed to the circadian shift.

Marijuana, CBD, and Cannabinoids

In all forms, medical marijuana (MMJ) is difficult to study, especially in children, because there are a range of doses, various ratios of CBD to THC, assorted preparations (gummy, other edibles, oil, vape), and different indications, from appetite to pain to insomnia to ASD-related self-injury. Not to mention, in most of the US, it's still illegal. MMJ might be helpful for neurodiverse kids, but how, how much, and for what? Adult studies have found small improvements in sleep coinciding with improvements in pain.[27] The research on the impact of MMJ on sleep in children and adolescents with ASD is inconsistent. Some studies show improvements in sleep, some show no improvements in sleep, and others show that sleep disruption can be a side effect of using MMJ for another condition![28] While anecdotally, MMJ might help some neurodiverse kids sleep better, it's important to consult a medical provider.

For additional information on MMJ for autism, the advocacy organization Hope Grows for Autism (www.hopegrowsforautism .org) offers education, recommended resources, and community support for families exploring MMJ.

Medications

Many people have used an antihistamine to see if it will help with sleep, for themselves or their children, and I'm one. Many, many parents have told me that their child's pediatrician suggested a few nights of diphenhydramine (Benadryl) to break the insomnia cycle. While antihistamines might have the beneficial side effect of sleepiness, it only takes a week or so to develop tolerance, thus the sleepiness advantage is short-lived. Antihistamines also have side effects, such as dry mouth, dizziness, constipation, cognitive slowing, and in rare cases, a paradoxical effect where kids are more energetic than ever. No, thank you.

There are no FDA-approved medications for insomnia in children, either over the counter or prescription. The FDA has approved extended-release sodium oxybate for children age seven and older who have narcolepsy, to treat cataplexy, or daytime sleepiness. Since sodium oxybate can be used for harmful purposes as a street drug (it's known as the "date rape drug"), this medicine is regulated out the wazoo. Don't even ask about it unless your child or teen has documented narcolepsy via a conclusive daytime nap study.

Off-Label Prescriptions

Even though there are no FDA-*approved* medications to help children fall asleep and stay asleep, there are certainly medications *used* for such purposes in neurodiverse children and teens.[29] In general, these medications have been FDA-approved for other uses in pediatrics, such as seizures, anxiety, or ADHD. But physicians can prescribe these "off-label," which is an extremely common practice with low-risk medications. Table 18.2 lists medications often prescribed in this way.

Clonidine, for example, is the most prescribed medication for sleep in children with neurodevelopmental conditions, and it has been used in pediatrics for more than fifty years. It is used to treat high blood pressure and ADHD, and it is even used for neonatal abstinence syndrome in the teeniest and youngest of babies. Other medications in this class of alpha-2 agonists are extended-release clonidine (Kapvay, Onyda) and extended-release guanfacine (Intuniv), which are FDA-approved in children for ADHD but not for sleep.[30] Although approved for seizures, restless legs syndrome, and nerve pain, GABA analogs such as gabapentin have been shown to be safe, well tolerated, and effective for some neurodiverse children and teens with sleep problems.[31]

The name "atypical antipsychotics" is horrible, but these medications can be helpful in reducing disruptive behaviors in children with neurodevelopmental and/or mental health conditions. Two such atypicals, aripiprazole and risperidone, are widely prescribed in neurodiverse children, and better sleep may be an added side effect.[32] These are rarely a first-line therapy for sleep because they can cause obesity and other side effects that may exacerbate sleep-disordered breathing and worsen obstructive sleep apnea. Benzodiazepines ("benzos") are also not first-choice medications in pediatrics despite a few small studies showing improved sleep in children with ASD or Williams syndrome. Lorazepam, diazepam, and clonazepam ("the pams") are benzodiazepines used in pediatrics for seizures, and they are sometimes prescribed off-label to treat periodic limb movement disorder and restless legs syndrome. While "benzos" have been prescribed for insomnia in adults for many years, there aren't many pediatric insomnia studies. Not only can they cause breathing difficulties, but they are more dangerous in terms of accidental ingestion, addiction, and overdose.

Several medications are approved for sleep in adults but not for children. Nonbenzodiazepine hypnotics, also known as the Z medications (zolpidem), have not been shown to improve sleep in children and teens, and they cause side effects, such as dizziness and headache. Children and adolescents also don't like how they feel, and the medications don't extend sleep time. Two newer medications approved for sleep in adults, ramelteon and suvorexant, act on melatonin receptors. They are promising, but they have not been well studied in pediatrics.

Trazodone, mirtazapine, and doxepin are older antidepressants with sedating side effects that are approved for insomnia in adults. Few studies have investigated their efficacy and side effects in neurodiverse children and adolescents, yet they are frequently used for children with insomnia and mood disorders. In fact, a study of psychiatrists in the US found that trazodone was the most prescribed sleep medication for adults and children with depression or anxiety.

Table 18.2: Off-Label Use of Medications to Improve Children's Sleep

Medication	FDA-approved uses
Antihistamines (diphenhydramine, hydroxyzine)	Approved for anxiety, allergies, and presurgical sleep in children age six and older.
Alpha 2 agonists (clonidine/ Kapvay, guanfacine/Onyda)	Extended-release approved for ADHD in children age six and older, regular-release not approved.
GABA analogs (gabapentin)	Approved in children age three and older for partial seizures.

Table 18.2: Off-Label Use of Medications to Improve Children's Sleep (*continued*)

Medication	FDA-approved uses
Antipsychotics (aripiprazole, risperidone)	Approved in children age five or older for irritability associated with ASD, depending on specific medication.
Benzodiazepines (diazepam, lorazepam, clonazepam)	Approved in children ages two to twelve for seizures, depending on specific medication.
Nonbenzodiazepine hypnotics (zolpidem)	Approved for sleep in adults.
Melatonin-receptor agonist (ramelteon, tasimelteon)	Approved for sleep in adults.
Orexin-receptor agonist (suvorexant)	Approved for sleep in adults.
Tricyclic antidepressant (doxepin)	Approved for sleep in adults.

The Extended-Release Problem

One problem with extended-release medications and supplements is that most of them must be swallowed whole (though liquid, extended-release clonidine hydrochloride, Onyda, is an exception), and pill swallowing can be difficult for children with neurodevelopmental conditions because of sensory issues, gag reflex, and anxiety. Many kids can swallow pills at about age five or six, though neurodiverse kids may take a bit longer.

I remember Henry learning to swallow pills. I once ordered

$54.91 of pill-swallowing aids. Henry was prescribed an extended-release tablet that had to be swallowed, and I was nervous, anticipating a tough time. I bought a few different special swallowing cups, strawberry-flavored mouth-glide spray, strawberry ice cream topping, applesauce, Jell-O, a bunch of candies of various sizes, and a pill box. On the first try, he took the medication from my palm with his fingers, stuck the pill in his mouth, swallowed it with one sip of water, and that was that.

PILL SWALLOWING TIPS

- If currently taking a liquid or chewable form of the medicine, try to practice pill swallowing before stopping the liquid. That way there is less pressure to master it quickly.
- Practice for five to ten minutes at a time at most. Give a small reward after each practice.
- Start with a sip of water or other beverage to get the mouth ready. Have your child start by swallowing small sprinkles, then move on to small candies like nerds, and gradually move up to mini M&Ms, Tic Tacs, and so on.
- If there is a setback one day and anxiety gets in the way, go back to the previous size and stay there for a few practices until your child is more confident.
- Place the pill on your child's tongue and have them take a sip of water but not swallow. Have them look down and put their chin to their chest and then swallow.
- Or: Use a straw. Place the pill far back on the tongue (not too far back or it will trigger the gag reflex) and have your child drink a favorite beverage through a straw.
- Or: Put the pill on a spoonful of applesauce, pudding, Jell-O, or chocolate syrup and have them swallow it.

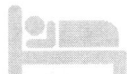

Tuck-In Tips

- Melatonin is the most researched medication or supplement used to improve the sleep of neurodiverse children and teens. Side effects are rare. Gummies are known to be unreliable in terms of the amount of melatonin.
- Iron supplements may be helpful if your child has trouble falling asleep due to restlessness *and* they have a low serum ferritin level. Supplementing with iron should be done under the guidance of a healthcare provider.
- There are not many studies about the effect of medical marijuana on children's sleep.
- There are no FDA-approved medications for insomnia in children. However, for decades, physicians have used "off-label" prescriptions of certain medications to improve sleep in neurodiverse kids.
- Most extended-release tablets must be swallowed; they cannot be chewed.

Pillow Point

While there is no magic pill to help with sleep, melatonin can have a positive impact on falling asleep in neurodivergent people.

Chapter 19

Nothing Is Working!
What Else Is There?

When I first started working as a licensed psychologist after eight years of post-undergraduate training, I saw a family that I still think about. Their toddler had frequent, severe tantrums and seemed to be on the move every moment of the day. This child's mom was on it. She was smart, she was an attorney, and she was just returning to work after being home with her son, who had been kicked out of multiple daycares and preschools. He was now attending a therapeutic preschool where he received speech and occupational therapy, and the situation was stable enough that this mom could finally go back to work.

The problem was that he still wasn't sleeping, and so she wasn't sleeping, which wasn't sustainable. According to the family, their pediatrician thought he probably had ADHD, but was uncomfortable prescribing stimulants to a child so young, and he started thinking way, way out of the box — so far out of the box that he was in another stratosphere. He recommended that the child, who was still drinking a bottle of milk at breakfast, be given Pepsi in the bottle instead, as a sort of improvised stimulant. When I imagine this, it makes my teeth hurt. While it's true that many kids with ADHD sleep better at night when they take daytime stimulant medication, I have never seen these results replicated with caffeinated cola in a preschool population. I was stunned, and I admit I was judgmental about this whole situation. Why on earth would anyone try this? As a new psychologist and not yet a parent, I didn't get it.

When nothing mainstream is working, sleep-deprived families turn to *anything* with even the tiniest possibility of improving sleep — including herbs, essential oils, water sounds, turkey as a bedtime snack, pig enzymes, and yes, Pepsi in a baby bottle. Regardless, I don't recommend giving toddlers Pepsi.

However, there's value in flexibility and trying new ideas if they aren't harmful or unhealthy, though personally, I'm more willing to experiment on myself than on my kids. This chapter surveys techniques and products that, according to anecdotal claims, have helped neurodiverse kids with sleep problems. None have been well researched, and I don't formally or officially recommend any of them. But it's good to know what other people have tried, and then decide for yourself if there's anything *you* want to try, and discuss it with a medical provider.

Did Pepsi solve the family's sleep issues? No. Improvement came because of the techniques I've already discussed: a consistent bedtime routine, a straightforward behavioral approach to bedtime, and a melatonin supplement. Along with these ingredients were two more: validation and support.

Diets and Dietary Supplements

There are many dietary supplements other than those discussed in chapter 18 that claim to improve sleep, almost like a magic wand. Ashwagandha, GABAdone, L-Carnitine, and valerian root supplements purportedly fix sleep problems, and it is possible that they might. But there aren't good scientific studies in adults or children demonstrating that these supplements are effective and, more importantly, safe.[1]

Neurodiverse kids and teens can be picky eaters. Nearly 70 percent of kids with ASD don't eat vegetables, and 25 percent don't eat fruit. The most common deficiencies (vitamins D and E, fiber, calcium, potassium, pantothenic acid, and choline) are usually not resolved with dietary supplements. These deficiencies have not been associated with restricted growth or obesity or with sleep in neurodiverse kids.[2] On the other hand, taking supplements has been associated with excess vitamin A, vitamin C, folate, zinc, copper, and manganese.[3]

The substances in table 19.1 purportedly improve sleep in humans, but there is minimal support in scientific journals, and I've seen zero good-quality studies on neurodiverse children or teens.[4] Does no research mean something won't help? No, but there isn't enough science yet for me to feel OK about giving it to my own kids. One low-risk option is to look for dietary sources of these substances, which are less likely to be harmful. If eating these foods helps your child or teen sleep better, that's great.

Table 19.1: Dietary Sources of Substances Reported to Improve Sleep

Supplement	Dietary sources
Vitamin B6	Meat, dairy, potatoes, bananas
Chamomile	Chamomile tea
Tart cherry	Tart cherry juice
Coenzyme Q10 (CoQ10)	Sesame seeds, pistachios, brown rice, spinach, broccoli, cauliflower, oranges
Vitamin D	Fish, dairy, egg yolks, mushrooms

Table 19.1: Dietary Sources of Substances Reported to Improve Sleep (*continued*)

Supplement	Dietary sources
Iron	Red meat, chicken thighs, green leafy veggies, beans
Melatonin	Mushrooms, kidney beans, pistachios
Magnesium	Pumpkin seeds, chia seeds, almond, spinach
Omega-3 fatty acids	Salmon, herring, sardines, trout
Potassium	Banana, legumes, nuts
Probiotics	Yogurt, kefir, kombucha
L-theanine	Green, white, and black tea
Tryptophan	Poultry, fish, egg whites, dairy, oats, flaxseed
Turmeric	Um, turmeric
Zinc	Meat, fish, dairy, eggs, oats, quinoa, brown rice, dark chocolate

Probiotics

Probiotics might improve the tummy troubles common in neuro-diverse children and teens; however, they haven't been shown to impact sleep in children with ADHD and/or ASD.[5] Similarly, anti-oxidant supplements such as CoQ10 may be beneficial for neuro-diverse kids in other ways, but when it comes to improving sleep, there isn't enough research in kids to recommend it.[6] If I wanted to increase my son's antioxidant levels with a supplement, I would probably give him melatonin, because it is the most well-studied antioxidant supplement in neurodiverse kids and teens.

Specialized Diets

People feel strongly about diets, kind of like they feel strongly about sleep. While eliminating foods containing gluten, casein, dairy, artificial food dyes, carbohydrates, or other elements may improve other body systems, there isn't *objective* evidence that any diet improves sleep in neurodiverse kids.[7] This means there isn't solid research using reliable and valid measures of sleep, such as a wearable sleep tracker or an overnight sleep study.

However, one study shows that parents of children with neurodevelopmental conditions (primarily ASD) *report* that changing to a specific way of eating has helped with falling asleep and/or staying asleep.[8] Almost a thousand parents were surveyed across the United States, and out of over twenty choices, there were seven specific diets that a percentage of parents endorsed as helping sleep. In the sample, 19 percent of parents reported the Feingold diet helped with falling asleep, and 15 percent said it helped with staying asleep. Only 10 to 11 percent of parents reported improvements in their child's sleep with the other six diets.

Here are the bare bones basics of those diets:

1. **Feingold:** Consume no artificial colors, flavors, or preservatives and minimal salicylates (a compound similar to aspirin that is found in almonds, apples, berries, grapes, oranges, peaches, cucumbers, pickles, and mint).
2. **Ketogenic:** Replace carbohydrates with high-fat foods and moderate protein to help the body burn fat for energy instead of glucose (ketosis). This diet can lower the frequency of seizures in children with epilepsy.
3. **Paleo:** Consume whole, unprocessed foods like our Paleolithic ancestors, and avoid any grains, legumes, dairy, or processed foods.

4. **Low sugar:** Reduce intake of both added and naturally occurring sugars as well as processed foods. Prioritize foods with a low glycemic index to help stabilize blood sugar.

5. **Gluten-free and/or casein-free:** Consume no wheat, barley, rye, and/or dairy products and make sure dairy replacements do not contain casein.

6. **Observation and elimination:** Watch for reflux, vomiting, or other gastrointestinal discomfort and eliminate associated foods.

7. **Healthy diet:** Consume vegetables, fruit, whole grains, and lean proteins. Avoid added sugar and saturated and trans fats.

While these diets are unlikely to improve sleep in neurodivergent kids and teens, eliminating certain foods from your family's diet is your family's decision. As someone who does not want to miss *anything* that could help my children, I've wanted to try these diets, but since I lack superpowers, I haven't been successful. Henry's preferred foods are fruits, vegetables, fish, and meat. The only carbohydrates he will eat are french fries, cinnamon-raisin bagels, and soft pretzels. He does have a vicious sweet tooth and loves lemon Oreos, any gummy candy, Skittles, and dried fruit, but he typically doesn't overeat them. Where the ideal meets our family's real is that we mostly eat at home and try to maintain a healthy diet.

Because You Like It

I like to smell a candle or an essential oil as much as anyone. However, there isn't a particular scent that has been found to improve sleep in scientific studies. Lavender, chamomile, sage, and other essential oils may not directly improve your child's sleep, but if they like the smell, that's reason enough to include it in a bedtime routine. That lavender spray may not give you an extra hour of sleep, but it may be calming, which is what a bedtime routine should be.

As I mentioned, a sense-based bedtime routine can promote calm before sleep. I don't have specific recommendations; it depends on your child's preferences. At bedtime (when I remember) I encourage my children to notice the taste of their watermelon toothpaste (gross), the coolness of their ice water, the softness of our dog's fur, the smell of the hand soap in our bathroom, and the sounds in their bedrooms and out in the hall. I do this not because it helps them sleep, but because they like it. Don't spend time or money making a lavender pillow thinking it will eliminate your child's night wakings, but if you and your child are fans of lavender pillows, go right ahead.

Staying with the sensory theme, there is a smidge of research in pediatrics showing that binaural beats promote relaxation in children undergoing surgery. I will not be trying that for surgery, but I wonder if it might help neurodiverse kids and teens with sleep. Binaural beats (aka brainwave entrainment) happen when sounds of different frequencies are played in each ear. Our brain creates a third tone (the difference of the two frequencies), which is said to promote sleep and relaxation. Is this true or woo-woo? There isn't enough research to say, but it's not off the table. If you and your child like the sound and it can be played consistently all night long, try it and see.

Beds, Sheets, Blankets, and Clothes

Special beds have not been shown to improve sleep in neurodiverse children and teens, either. These often-expensive beds fall broadly into two categories: safety beds and sensory beds. Safety beds include enclosed beds (such as zip-up beds or tent beds), floor beds that no one can fall out of, and even cribs for younger children. I can't endorse any bed in terms of safety or effectiveness, but there are a lot of pricey options.

Other beds provide sensory input by vibrating or mimicking a baby's movement in the uterus, or simulating a parent rocking back and forth, bouncing up and down, or moving in an arc. There isn't good scientific research to show that consumer versions of these beds improve sleep, either. My impression is that parental sleep deprivation, anxiety, and desperation are driving this market, but I'm open to changing my mind if I see studies showing improved sleep. There are also slings, swings, and hammocks. Do not use any of these for infants or children with muscle weakness, as these positions can interfere with breathing.

Other than the bed itself, there are different kinds of sheets, blankets, and garments that claim to help neurodiverse kids sleep better. Several kids I've worked with love stretchy, Lycra sheets, while others have felt too confined or too hot. Sleeping bags have similar pros and cons. Research on weighted blankets is mixed in terms of improving sleep, but if your older child or teen likes the pressure or the feeling of a weighted blanket, go for it.[9] There are also compression garments (socks, sleeves, shirts) that may help children participate and engage in occupational therapy, but they have not been shown to help sleep.[10] Another item many parents find helpful is the sensory body sock. This is a large, stretchy sack that allows a child to fully extend their arms and legs. It usually zips or buttons, with the head left out, and it can be used for stretching and gentle resistance. In addition, seamless clothing options — such as socks, underwear, bras, and T-shirts — can make a big difference for kids and teens who are sensitive to seams.

As parents of neurodiverse kids, we often need to be creative and stray from the typical path. Still, I encourage you to do your own sleuthing and read reviews somewhere other than the company's website. Just recently, I almost spent fifty dollars on a vibrating egg that promised to make 100 percent of neurodiverse kids sleep through the night. Even I got sucked in and started thinking maybe it would help Henry's sleep. Then I looked for scientific studies (zero) and checked out reviews of the product on various websites other than the company's — and everyone who reviewed this vibrating egg said their neurodiverse child or teen hated it and it made sleep worse!

Acupuncture

Traditional Chinese medicine, primarily acupuncture, is used widely across conditions in adults, and it is being used more and more in pediatrics for headaches, postsurgical pain and nausea, cerebral palsy, Tourette syndrome, spinal cord injury, and even ADHD.[11] In terms of sleep problems, a few mediocre studies have looked at whether acupuncture helps insomnia,[12] but no rigorous studies have been done in either adults or children. A few promising studies support the use of acupuncture for bed-wetting as well as for the pain and nausea related to adenotonsillectomy (surgical removal of the tonsils and adenoids) for obstructive sleep apnea.[13] Additionally, acupuncture in combination with medication has been used to improve attention and concentration in kids and teens with ADHD, and this combination has been shown in one study to slightly improve sleep.[14]

Biofeedback and Neuromodulators

Biofeedback and neuromodulators are promising, but they are not standard treatment for pediatric sleep problems. Biofeedback encompasses techniques that help people change something in their bodies using feedback from a machine. I teach breathing and muscle relaxation with the goal of slowing down the person's heart rate, but I don't have a heart monitor that shows them when it is working, which would be biofeedback. A specific kind of biofeedback called neurofeedback involves learning to change brainwaves to promote relaxation and emotion regulation. In my experience, regardless of the impact on sleep, kids enjoy virtual reality and video games enough that they might be motivated to return for another session.

Neuromodulators excite or inhibit nerve pathways. They can be noninvasive (outside the body) or invasive (implanted in the body), and they can be in the form of medications, light, electrical stimulation (trigeminal nerve stimulation, TNS), or magnetic stimulation (transcranial magnetic stimulation, TMS). Strengthening or inhibiting nerve pathways is thought to promote the brain's ability to change, adapt, and correct miscommunication between different parts of the brain. In TNS and TMS, electrical or magnetic currents go through the skull to the brain temporarily. These treatments do not work instantly, and most studies of TNS and TMS involve using the device daily for a period of several weeks. Despite not being instantly effective, one benefit of a neuromodulator is that it can be removed and/or reversed without serious, permanent consequences. Most studies of TNS and TMS devices that claim to improve sleep have been in adults, though there are currently a few applications for older children and adolescents.

One example of targeted electrical nerve stimulation is a hypoglossal nerve stimulator for obstructive sleep apnea (OSA, which I describe in chapter 5). Activation of this nerve prevents the muscles that keep the airway open from collapsing during sleep, thus preventing OSA. This device is implanted under the skin.

Other noninvasive TNS devices use electrodes placed on the skin that are connected to a controller. When turned on, the electrodes deliver a small electrical current that travels to the brain. In addition to TNS improving ADHD symptoms, at least one study also found an increase in total sleep time and a decrease in night wakings.[15]

Transcranial magnetic stimulation can target nerve cells in the areas of the brain related to sleep. TMS is associated with parent-reported improvements in sleep, such as a shorter time to fall asleep and fewer and shorter night wakings.[16] Some scientists think that sensory abnormalities, specifically touch and hearing, relate to increased arousal and to GABA dysfunction.[17] TMS may improve sleep by altering these sensory abnormalities. In adults with insomnia, multiple studies have concluded that TMS is "safe and effective either alone or in combination with other treatments," but this research has not been done yet with children.[18]

Medications can also be neuromodulators, impacting messengers in the nervous system, such as neurotransmitters and neuropeptides. The main sleep-related neuropeptide is orexin (hypocretin), which has been implicated in narcolepsy. Other examples of neuromodulators include light exposure (alters circadian cells), certain antidepressants (alter neurotransmitters such as serotonin), and soundwaves.[19]

Research Participation

Every cure starts somewhere, and scientific research is the starting line. Participating in research might expose your child to something new that improves sleep, or it might not benefit you or your child at all. I decide what techniques to use in my practice based on scientific studies that are published in peer-reviewed journals. These studies are much more rigorous than what you might see online in a magazine, newspaper, or blog or on TikTok. To be published in a reputable scientific journal, before the study even starts, it must first be reviewed and approved by a hospital or university review board to make sure the study ethics are sound and risks to patients are minimal. After it is approved, the researcher does the study, the data is collected and analyzed, and the researcher considers the implications of the results. To share findings, the researcher writes a paper about their study and submits it to a journal that specializes in that particular area. The journal editor reviews it and sends the article to two to four anonymous volunteer experts in the field. Let me reassure you that nobody is getting any money to write or review these articles; I know from personal experience. The reviews are put together and sent back to the researcher with suggestions for revising the paper. The researcher must make each change or say why they didn't make the change, and then the paper is reviewed *again* at least once. One reason I trust research published in these kinds of journals is that I know how rigorous the process is.

Unfortunately, people who are not employed by a hospital or university typically don't have access to these types of journals. In that case, the journal tells you to contact the researcher to get a copy of the article, which may or may not work. Once you have the article in your hands, you might not be trained to gauge the quality of the study. This has nothing to do with intelligence, perseverance, thoroughness, or will. It is 100 percent about knowing what to evaluate. I have eight years of post-undergraduate training, and I still have to read each study a few times before I absorb all the details and can decide whether the study is good enough to believe the results.

Research also shows us when something is not helpful. Imagine that a small, early study of something shows promise for improving sleep in ten adults. The study must be done again (and again) in bigger, more diverse samples with comparison groups using stringent research methods. At this point, results often fall apart. This happened with digestive enzymes from pigs. Yes, you read that correctly. Porcine secretin once showed promise for improving sleep in very small samples of children with ASD.[20] More, bigger, and better studies unquestionably found that digestive enzymes from pigs don't help neurodivergent kids sleep better after all. Despite the failed pig experiment, from my perspective as a mom and as a sleep psychologist, there is almost always something to try next.

Tuck-In Tips

- Research published in reputable scientific journals is rigorous, which is one reason I look to science as my general guide.
- Parents of neurodivergent kids often think outside the box, which includes considering treatments without the strongest research foundation. This is OK as long as supplements, diets, and techniques are not harmful or unhealthy.
- Treatments with minimal research support that may or may not help sleep include acupuncture and neuromodulation devices.
- Existing research does not show that scents, blankets, or special beds help sleep. But it's OK to try something just because you or your child like it, as long as it's safe.

Pillow Point

I suggest first trying to improve your child's sleep by following the steps covered so far in part 2; however, it's OK to try things outside the box to improve your child's sleep, as long as they are safe and healthy.

Chapter 20

Teen Sleep Is a Different Animal

In one of the training clinics I supervised at the sleep center, I saw an unforgettable sixteen-year-old boy named Barry with a rare genetic condition called Prader-Willi syndrome. Barry had cognitive impairment, short stature, and an insatiable appetite, which are all common for people with his condition. He seemed to be both a teenager and a young child at the same time. He had difficulty both falling asleep and returning to sleep, and he had some anxiety about sleep that seemed to fit a straightforward insomnia diagnosis.

I explained to Barry and his mom that we needed to retrain Barry's brain that the bed is only for sleeping. That means it's not a good idea to be awake in bed for long periods of time. In addition to doing homework, eating, playing video games, or watching TV in bed, even lying in bed awake doing nothing still messes up the brain's association between the bed and sleep. So my usual recommendation is that when it feels like it's been about twenty or thirty minutes (don't look at the clock, just guess), get out of bed and do something neutral or boring (but not electronics). Usually I problem-solve with the family to decide what boring thing the teen will do. I gave Barry some examples that other teens have successfully used: reading old *Sports Illustrated* magazines, folding and unfolding the same basket of laundry, coloring or drawing, reading a history book, doing math problems, and reviewing the lyrics of favorite songs. None of these felt right, and Barry and his mom decided to figure it out when they got home.

About a month later, Barry came in for a follow-up visit. Since I had a trainee with me that day, I sent Paul in first to assess how Barry was doing. When he finished, Paul came out to spill the tea to the sleep team. According to Paul, both Barry and his mom reported that sleep had improved a lot. Barry had less bedtime anxiety and was falling asleep within thirty minutes. He was still getting out of bed a few times per week, but this was much better than a few times per night. Paul said that Barry had started writing poetry as the neutral boring thing he'd chosen to do when he couldn't sleep, and he was keeping a poetry journal. I was happily surprised.

Paul and I went back into the room together, and I talked about next steps with Barry and his mom. Near the end of the visit, I wanted to let Barry know how cool it was that he was writing poetry. I talked about how poetry can affect people, about how few poets there are, and I briefly mentioned my favorite poem, "One Art" by Elizabeth Bishop. I asked if he shared his poetry with any friends, and Barry shook his head. I sympathized, "Yeah, I can understand wanting to keep your writing to yourself. Middle schoolers aren't always into poetry." Barry gave me a slight smile.

I told him that I always loved to hear good ideas so that I could share them with other kids. I asked, "So tell me about your poetry. What do you like to write about?"

Barry answered with two words: "Dirty poetry."

Huh?

"You know, like dirty poetry," he repeated.

I looked at his mother, who had a hand over her eyes and was slowly shaking her head. I again asked Barry to clarify.

"You know, dirty like the birds and the bees."

Whoa. I was speechless. Barry's mom was now quietly laughing. My brain was literally void of any therapeutic response. I stammered out a few words about safety, creativity, and following your bliss, while making sure your bliss is respectful to others. Paul was trying to stay professional and keep it cool, but the wobbly, surprised O of his mouth and his wide eyes broadcast loud and clear that he was totally freaked out. Thank goodness Barry's mom came to the rescue. She assured us that she read his poems and was monitoring their content. She clarified that Barry's poems were mostly about the places he would take his girlfriend if he had one. You know, Chuck E. Cheese, Olive Garden, the park, or a movie like *Wreck-It Ralph* or *Moana*. Once in a while, the poems involved hand-holding or the occasional kiss, and she would joke with him, "Don't you be writing any of that dirty stuff."

Ah, *that* kind of dirty poetry. Whew.

Debunking the Myths About Teen Sleep

I owe my career to teenagers. As a graduate student, I loved working with teens, who were confused, grumpy, angsty, funny, cool, difficult, emotional, stoic, smart, you name it. Perhaps because my own teenage years were such a prickly time of life, I love connecting with kids navigating the jungle of adolescence. When it was time to finalize my dissertation topic, I decided that I wanted my research to make a big impact on adolescent health. I looked up the leading causes of medical problems and death in teenagers. Then as now, the top three are accidents, homicide, and suicide. They are each very different, but all relate to sleep. At night, and in the context of disrupted sleep, decision making ability is impaired, impulsivity may be increased, and mood is at its lowest, increasing the risk for all three. Of course, other factors are in play, but the issue of sleep stole my heart, and I decided to focus my research on the incredibly important and fascinating topic of adolescent sleep.

Of course, I had no idea that years later the reverse would be true: My heart (my children) would steal my sleep!

The first thing I noticed was the multitude of sleep myths

shared by adolescents, their parents, and our whole society. For example, sleepiness is often mischaracterized as laziness, when really adolescent biology plus early school start times create the lion's share of sleep-deprived adolescents.

Let's call out some other myths about teenage sleep:[1]

- It's better to stay up late studying for a test than it is to get more sleep.
- Adolescents can't control their sleep schedules.
- Caffeine, energy drinks, and other stimulants counteract the impacts of sleep deprivation.
- Naps after school are fine if nighttime sleep is poor.
- A later bedtime and wake time on weekends is OK, if you get the right amount of sleep.
- Adolescents need much less sleep than school-age children.

All of these myths are false. What's the truth? Let's review what the science says:

A large body of research shows that puberty causes natural, normal biological changes to circadian rhythms that affect sleep and sleepiness considerably. No matter which of the seven continents teenagers live on, they experience a circadian delay of about two hours. The sleepiness an eight-year-old feels at 8 p.m. happens around 10 p.m. or later for a thirteen-year-old, but school starts at the same time regardless of bedtime. The impact of later school start times is significant, and the American Academy of Pediatrics officially recommends middle and high schools start no earlier than 8:30 a.m. This recommendation is wonderful…when it is followed. In the three school districts our family has been part of, there is a work-around: period 0. The first academic period starts at 8:30 a.m., but teens may "choose" to start school as early as 7 a.m. if they want an elective like art, music, or STEM. Neurodiverse students often must use their elective periods for occupational therapy, speech therapy, tutoring, or study skills, so if they want to take a fun elective, they have to start school with period o. Students who arguably need sleep the most, have more learning challenges, *and* have the most sleep problems are supposed to wake up the earliest. Hmmm.

Research also shows that factors such as an earlier parent-set bedtime, physical activity, and good sleep hygiene relate to a shorter time to fall asleep and more overall sleep.[2] On the flip side, family conflict, evening light exposure, tobacco, caffeine, and the use of some electronics for some teens relate to later bedtimes, longer time to fall asleep, and less total sleep time.

Dr. Beth Malow recently found that the sleep schedules of teenagers with ASD may not follow the pattern of later bedtimes, decreased sleep duration, and increased sleepiness that is characteristic of neurotypical teenagers.[3] In her study, which followed the same children over several years, elementary-aged children had similar bedtimes whether they had ASD or not. As those same children approached puberty, the neurotypical teens developed later bedtimes and were sleepier, while the bedtimes and sleepiness of teens with ASD stayed the same, likely due to parents being more involved in nighttime schedules. Wake times for both groups were similar over time (probably due to school start times), which suggests that, for a few years at least, neurodiverse teens might get more sleep than their neurotypical peers.

What Bedroom Routine Do Teens Want?

When neurodiverse adolescents were asked, "What makes a good night's sleep for you?" They identified some common elements both at night and during the day that help sleep.[4] First, independence and agency over the activities that happen before bedtime and during the bedtime routine were strong catalysts for good sleep. While it was helpful for parents to provide some guidance, teens wanted to choose their own pre-sleep routines, especially the sensory elements.

For these neurodiverse adolescents, the right level and kind of sensory input were critical influences on the ease of falling asleep and staying asleep as well as self-perceived quality of sleep. Sensory preferences and familiarity in terms of foods (bedtime snack), materials (pajamas, sheets, and bedclothes), smells (room, laundry soap), sounds (soothing and consistent), temperature (of the room and themselves), and light (just right) were identified as key determinants of sleep. For example, adolescents reported that a specific, favorite, predictable bedtime snack (in terms of taste, texture, color, and temperature) helped them to calm down.

Additional elements they identified as promoting good sleep occur at specific times of day, as follows:

After Dinner and Before Bedtime

- Time with family being close, but not too close (watching a TV show, reading side by side, playing a board game with clear rules and without intense competition), and keeping conversation light, easy, and short, with no end goal.
- Uninterrupted time with familiar, focused interests, including activities, objects, or even thoughts.
- Having no structured evening activities at all led to the best bedtimes (by their report).

Bedtime Routine

- A custom bedtime routine that is specifically for them, even if it breaks normal sleep hygiene rules, so parents should be flexible. (For more about this, see chapter 11.)
- Adolescents know their preferred sensory experiences. Cold fruit, crunchy pretzels, or soft string cheese might be a good bedtime snack.
- After stressful parts of the routine, such as washing face,

body, and hair as well as brushing teeth, time to calm down is needed. Familiarity and repetition help to regulate and reset the body and mind. Fidgets, stress balls, videos, music, books, and dialogue from movies and shows can relieve stress.

- A hug or pat from a parent as well as other familiar shared rituals — like taking turns listing state capitals, naming animal characteristics, or hearing well-known songs — are comforting.

Waiting for Sleep

- Mentally reviewing plans for the next day.
- Occupying the mind with the details of particular things, like Pokémon characters, features of the solar system, or a favorite baseball player's statistics.
- Meditation, breathing, and muscle relaxation.

Daytime Factors That Make Bedtime Easier

- Daytime physical activity like walking, jogging, swimming, or biking outside of school (not PE class).
- Uninterrupted time doing favorite activities that include a balance of easy and hard.
- A routine way of thinking about and handling interesting objects or details.
- Feeling calm and happy.
- Connecting with a teacher, a favorite class, an activity in school that day, or having something to look forward to at school.

I had a lightbulb moment when I read all this — especially about family time that is close but not too close and the importance of things that are familiar and repetitive at bedtime. At first I thought the aha was that I learned some new things that might make Henry's sleep better, but then I realized it was about me. Henry is not alone in his quirky nighttime preferences, and those are not because of something I've done wrong as a mom. Neurodiverse teens everywhere like to end their days with the expected snack, the usual big hug from a parent, the dependable phrase ("Have a good sleep!"), and/or the same song before closing their eyes.

Reconciling ideal sleep standards with respect for agency and independence involves negotiation and compromise on everyone's part. I've been most successful in negotiating healthy sleep behaviors with adolescents by using a good, better, best approach. It's another way to conceptualize the intersection of the ideal and the real. In chapter 5, I tell the story of Daysha and her CPAP. Eventually, Daysha agreed to wear her CPAP every day except when she had Friday sleepovers with friends. "Best" would have been wearing her CPAP every night, but agreeing to one night off was "better" than wearing it five nights per week. "Good" might have been agreeing to use it four nights per week.

Sleep space is another example. The desire for more alone time is both part of adolescence and part of being neurodiverse. For most youth, alone time occurs in their bedroom, and sometimes the only comfy spot is their bed. However, the ideal is to use the bed only for sleeping; that's "best." But if the bed is your teen's only option for hanging out in their room, then "better" is finding ways to differentiate your teen's sleep space from their hangout space. When chilling on the bed, perhaps they could use a separate pillow, always stay on top of the blanket, face a different direction, and stay sitting up. "Good" might be sitting up with a separate pillow, but being under the covers.

Here are more good, better, best examples related to elements of sleep:

Table 20.1: Good, Better, Best with Sleep Routines

	Good	Better	Best
Stimulating activities before bed	Switch from YouTube, social media, and video games to a familiar movie or TV show.	Watch a familiar movie or TV show outside of bed. Turn off electronics before getting into bed.	No electronics once bedtime routine starts.
Light	Parents turn teen's overhead light off when they go to bed.	Dim overhead light at teen's bedtime.	Use a nightlight instead.
Phone/iPad	Use the phone/iPad as an alarm, but keep under bed.	Switch to an alarm clock and charge devices across the room.	Use an alarm clock and charge devices in another room.
Naps	Shorten nap to thirty minutes and wake daily by 4:30 p.m. Sleep late on weekends.	Eliminate nap but sleep late on weekends.	Keep a schedule on weekends within two hours of weekday schedule. No naps.
Sound	Listen to loud, energetic songs while playing air guitar on the bed.	Listen to calming music sitting on a beanbag near the bed.	Listen to continuous sound machine or white noise overnight.

Table 20.1: Good, Better, Best with Sleep Routines (*continued*)

	Good	Better	Best
Sleep space	Fall asleep on couch watching TV.	Fall asleep in comfy chair in own bedroom.	Fall asleep in own bed.
Caffeine	Drink coffee in the morning and soda after school.	Drink coffee in the morning and soda no later than lunch.	Switch to decaf coffee and soda.

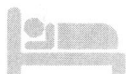

Tuck-In Tips

- Near puberty, adolescents develop a biological two-hour delay in their circadian rhythm.
- Keep a consistent, daily bedtime and wake-time schedule (no more than two hours later on non-school days).
- Avoid all daytime sleep and avoid caffeine after lunch.
- Use a good, better, best approach when negotiating healthy sleep habits with your teen.
- Be flexible where you can with bedtime routines. Adolescents want to choose their nighttime activities and often prefer the familiar and repetitive.

Pillow Point

Discuss ideal sleep habits with your teen and collaborate when determining a bedtime routine and setting realistic goals for improving sleep.

Chapter 21

What About the Rest
of the Family?

Strangely, while I was finishing this book, I had a similar con-versation with two different friends about how we *must* stay alive forever because our neurodiverse children need us to function. Not that our children need help in general but that they need *our* help specifically. One friend told me that at her annual gy-necological visit, she asked about getting a preventative bilateral mastectomy so that she could at least cross one thing — breast cancer — off the list of things that could kill her. It might sound extreme, but I thought it was genius. I've decided to ask my doctor about that and see if she could take out the ovaries and uterus, too, while I'm already under anesthesia.

If your neurodiverse child is on track to becoming an inde-pendent adult, you might not worry about living forever. Talking with my friend reassured me that other parents of neurodiverse kids have the same fear. What will happen to our children when we are no longer here to protect and take care of them? After we talked about living forever, I told her that I'd had a donut and two cups of coffee for dinner. I also hadn't exercised for months due to spending every extra minute with my kids because I was feel-ing guilty about the time I was spending at work and writing this book. Exercise is probably the most important, changeable thing I can do to live a longer life, yet I rarely feel justified taking the time to play tennis or take a Pilates class.

Another friend who was an early reader of this book asked me how the heck I was finding the time to write it. The truth is not very healthy. For about nine months, I went to the office many Saturdays, leaving home at 5 or 6 a.m., wrote all day, and came back just in time for dinner and my kids' bedtime. My husband and my mom graciously picked up the slack. In addition, six times I spent the night in a hotel. I drank coffee, tea, and/or diet Coke nonstop while writing until the wee hours of the morning. Then I crashed, slept for a few hours, and wrote again until checkout. If you are reading this, apparently it worked out.

Self-Care for Sleep-Deprived Parents

Clearly, I'm no expert on self-care. Actually, I think self-preservation is a more accurate term when it comes to sleep-deprived parents of neurodiverse kids. To me, prioritizing self-care is like trying to relax and drink a cup of hot tea while simultaneously playing whack-a-mole. We all know we should exercise, eat healthy, get eight hours of sleep per night, and floss our teeth daily for optimal well-being. How many of us do that consistently? I don't. Personally, I need the CliffsNotes version of self-care, and maybe you do, too. From my perspective, it comes down to six key categories. Some focus on smaller, simpler ways to recharge, and some are essential aspects of mental and emotional well-being.

Community and Unity

I say it over and over because I think finding your people is essential. First, it means building the team that helps care for your child, but it also means gathering the people who help take care of you.

For me, that means my friends (mostly my mom friends) who

span different stages of my life. As one example, my best friend of thirty years has made even the briefest reunions possible, starting before Simon was born. Twice a year on our birthdays we meet for lunch in a town halfway between us (about an hour away). Those lunches are a lifeline. We savor yummy food while trying to remember titles of recent books we've read, laughing our heads off, sharing stories from our jobs and families, and sometimes hashing out solutions to whatever dilemmas are happening in our lives. We talk about fantasy futures, like starting a foundation to help families with neurodiverse kids find services, buying a huge mansion to help young mothers in foster care, or selling our houses for double the price and retiring on the beach. Over the years, reading glasses have become essential, and our memories have gotten a little fuzzier, but the connection has never wavered.

Of course, the ideal isn't always possible. Life is busy, and sometimes we can't meet people in person as much as we'd like. That's OK. The important thing is to connect as much as you can for as long as you can with the people who make you feel good. That might mean texting a friend rather than visiting, grabbing coffee with a work friend, or even consistently shopping at neighborhood stores where the people are friendly and know you.

I believe we can experience support and community from interacting with all living things. Don't overlook the power of pets. I have always loved my pets so much that it teeters on the edge of unhealthy. Right now, we have one dog, and simply petting her, rubbing her tummy, or sitting with her gives me a sense of love and well-being. Taking care of plants, tending to a garden, or just walking outside in nature are other ways to feel connected. I also recommend getting as much sunlight as possible. Even small doses, especially in the morning, can lift mood and improve sleep.

Tonglen is a meditation and breathing practice that fosters connection on a spiritual or emotional level (see chapter 17). I practice my own approximation of it, which probably shouldn't even be called Tonglen, but this practice helps me feel less alone and more connected. Some find meditation too "woo-woo," but I find it powerful.

While I mostly read for entertainment, in the service of book research, I finally read Kate Swenson's book *Forever Boy*, and I was stunned. I can't even describe how I felt reading words that seemed to be written about *me* by a person I don't even know in a completely different situation. I have a lot of support from friends and family, but realizing that this neurodiverse parenting journey comes with thoughts and feelings unique to us has been transformative. On the surface, nothing has changed. I still don't exercise enough. I let my kids watch too many screens. I don't drink enough water. I buy too many things on the internet. Inside, though, something has shifted.

There is a part of having a neurodiverse child with sleep problems that is both unique and lonely. Kate writes that this isolation is "the kind of lonely that comes from knowing in your heart that your child is different and there is nothing you can do to change it. It's a loneliness that creeps in at 3 a.m. after being awake for hours with a screaming child, wondering why they won't sleep." Even if you have great social support, it is life-changing to connect with people who have similar struggles. Reading, listening to, and watching the stories of others can foster connection and be good self-care.

Religion, Spirituality, Meditation

For many people, some form of religion, spirituality, or meditation is a fundamental part of identity and community. These practices can bring balance, structure, meaning, and comfort to the daily struggles and successes we all experience. For parents of neurodivergent children, attending a quiet, formal service in a church, synagogue, mosque, temple, or other sacred space can feel impossible. When our attention is on our child, or on anticipating their needs, it can be hard to fully engage in a sermon, teaching, or ritual. Instead, spiritual or meditation practice might take simpler, more flexible forms: reading a short passage from a sacred or inspirational text, offering a brief prayer at bedtime, or pausing for five minutes of mindfulness. While I would love to go on a weeklong silent meditation retreat, I often settle for a few deep breaths. Religious, spiritual, and contemplative practices, in whatever form, can be a key part of self-preservation.

Connecting to the Present Moment

A very effective way to bring yourself into the present moment is to focus your attention on something sensory. I'm pretty attuned to smells (for better or worse), and so I choose products that smell good to me when I engage in the various happenings of the day. I shower with my favorite coconut soap, use jasmine-scented deodorant, and prefer a face sunscreen that faintly smells like roses. I use sage-scented hand soap in one bathroom and lilac in the other. My laundry detergent is bergamot and magnolia, and my dish soap is peony. This probably sounds like an overwhelming perfumatorium of jumbled smells, but it works for me. Another thing I savor and enjoy is eating Brown Cow maple yogurt. Until last year, I only ate it rarely because it is full fat (the horror!). Then I decided that the pleasure of eating it far outweighs the few extra calories. Sometimes I treat myself to an iced matcha from my local coffee shop because they have the good (nugget) ice. I've noticed that kids appreciate small things, too. When they touch or hear something they love, many of my patients often say, "That's so satisfying." I keep a variety of fidgets in my office, and I keep getting more because watching kids light up when they find the one that feels so perfectly satisfying is also satisfying to me.

Entertainment and Distraction

Distracting ourselves through entertainment can also be a form of self-preservation. Options might include music, movies, and shows; games, from pickleball to Wordle, softball to Scrabble, Candy Crush to whatever new app exists; and of course, books and reading. All these things can help us take our minds somewhere else. Reading is my go-to. I usually use the Kindle app on my phone, so even five spare minutes at the pharmacy becomes reading time. Poems or articles in *The New York Times* or *People* also fit into the nooks and crannies of my day. Podcasts are another favorite; commuting is my time to enjoy a gripping true-crime story.

Usually, I tend to avoid media focused on neurodiversity, and I'm not 100 percent sure why. While my friends tell me that the TV series *Love on the Spectrum* and *The Good Doctor* are excellent, I haven't watched them yet. I don't usually read memoirs or blogs about neurodiverse parenting, either. The one exception is Kate Swenson's pioneering blog *Finding Cooper's Voice*, which I have read intermittently over the years. Sometimes it has been a lifeline, and other times, it's too close to home and just painful, so I go back to entertainment and fashion blogs. However, while writing this book, I realized I could now read books and blogs written by neurodiverse parents without a tightness in my chest and a sick stomach. I feel like I've made progress.

Managing Overload for Mental Health

One of the most important tasks for parents is managing overload. Parenting a neurodiverse child can feel heavy, and at times, the demands can be overwhelming. Avoiding overwhelm is a crucial aspect of caring for your mental health. While I am a psychologist, I don't believe therapy is mandatory for everyone. But talking to someone outside of your situation whose job it is to listen and support you can be incredibly valuable. A therapist can help you manage stress, worry, sadness, complicated relationships, anger, and everything in between.

Sometimes we get trapped in our own minds. Feeling isolated

or different can lead us to create this protective bubble, but inside it, we might develop thoughts and beliefs about ourselves that are critical, harsh, or downright mean. We might not even notice these patterns until we feel depressed, anxious, overwhelmed, or overloaded. Talking to a psychologist, therapist, or counselor can help transform these thoughts to be more helpful, encouraging, and functional. Even if you can't change your situation, therapy can help you adjust, cope, and be more compassionate to yourself.

Unfortunately, parents of neurodiverse children do not always find their way to mental health providers. One study showed that about half (54.3 percent) of parents of kids with neurodevelopmental conditions accessed mental health services in the previous year.[1] The most common reasons for not doing so weren't surprising: lack of time and lack of appropriate childcare. One thing that isn't on most people's radar is that parents of neurodiverse kids can't always just "get a sitter." Appropriate childcare can mean needing people with training and experience with children like your child. It can mean managing a feeding tube, elopement, or aggression. The average high school kid doesn't have this experience. Since the Covid pandemic, online therapy has become widespread. Several studies have shown that remote virtual therapy is as good as or better than in-person therapy for treating adults with depression.[2] Studies also show that internet-delivered therapy for parents of neurodiverse children with sleep problems can be effective.[3]

Managing overload is primarily about mental health, but it can also be about the sheer number of things we have to do every day. I was just at a conference for mothers of children with autism, and several women talked about the benefits of outsourcing. While parents have to do many things related to their neurodiverse child, plenty of unrelated things *don't* need to be done by a parent — like grocery shopping, laundry, and cleaning. Some women paid for these kinds of services, and some traded with other parents. Most of them described feeling guilty about outsourcing, but they also recognized the positive impact of not doing everything themselves.

Routines and Checklists

Routines can also ease your mental load and give you a sense of accomplishment. For example, I read every night before bed, and no matter what else happened that day, I know I've read (for my own self-care). Building in a gratitude practice, whether through journaling or simply pausing to reflect, can also highlight the things you've achieved. Have gratitude for yourself. And don't underestimate the power of checklists. They aren't just for neurodiverse kids! Not only can they help us stay organized, but they also give us a tangible way to recognize and acknowledge what we've done.

The Rest of the Family's Sleep

I generally use science as my north star, but research on the caregivers of neurodiverse children can sometimes be just so *duh* and *ugh*. When the child has less sleep, the parent has less sleep and more daytime stress.[4] Really? We need another study to confirm that? I already live it!

In fact, of the hundreds of studies of sleep and neurodivergence, very few investigate parent or sibling sleep, but it's no surprise that stress relates to poor sleep in parents of neurodiverse kids. And it's not just how parents *feel* about their sleep; it's their objectively measured sleep.[5] One study showed that not only do parents rate their sleep quality as worse, but they wake up about forty-five minutes earlier and get about forty minutes less sleep each night. They are also less likely to take sleep medications, which doesn't surprise me at all. Since I've had Henry and Simon, I try not to do anything that would prevent me from going to the emergency room at 2 a.m. if needed.

Nor is it just the sleep disruptions from a child's night wakings that cause poor parental sleep.[6] It's the stress! And the guilt! As parents, most of us have guilt, but for many years I sort of welcomed its steady presence. I rationalized that guilt was good because it kept me remembering and prioritizing the right things and prevented me from leaving any stone unturned. Yet it's horrible for mental health. The strongest predictors of anxiety and depression in parents of neurodiverse children are poor sleep and guilt.[7] I love it when science and real life come together.

On the flip side, research also finds that parents of neurodiverse kids are happy, resilient, and have both new and enduring friendships.[8] Good for us! I sometimes worry that this book makes parenting neurodiverse kids sound devoid of joy, and that's not true by a long shot. It's not true for me or for any of my friends with neurodiverse kids. One of the things that has surprised me over the years is how little my son's neurodiversity impacts my parenting happiness. I experience a boatload of worry, a lot of work, and a lack of sleep, *and* I feel a whole lot of joy. In fact, sometimes I wish I still had that damn "JOY" sweater!

Siblings

Our complicated hearts worry and break for our neurotypical children, too. As I worked on this book, the thought kept popping into my head that, to Simon, this book might be further evidence that Henry is my favorite child. It's so hard to explain that the extra attention, time, appointments, rule bending, and cookies at bedtime are not because Henry is my favorite. Both of my sons are my favorite, of course. Not being able to listen to the radio on the way to school or having to eat at home instead of at a restaurant is not because I will do anything Henry wants. It's because I am trying to keep *everyone* safe and comfortable. Personally, I'd love to listen to the radio.

Especially when siblings are young, it's hard to talk about neurodivergence in a neutral way. When Simon was three, I was dropping Henry off at a summer camp for neurodivergent kids, and Simon yelled to the counselors, "Hey guys, next summer when I have autism, I'll be coming to this camp, too!" Simon used to view the various therapies I took Henry to as a special, fun time with Mom that he didn't get. Before Simon started kindergarten, I did not work on Fridays so that the two of us, and only us, could have "adventure day." The adventure might have been going to the supermarket, the park, or the zoo, but nonetheless it was time for just me and Simon. I remind him of that today, and I still let him sleep in my bed probably once a week. In fact, my friends used to jokingly call me "the faux sleep doctor," since by day I helped other kids learn to sleep on their own but at night I let Simon sleep in my bed. Once in a blue moon when Simon is almost asleep, I'll whisper, "You're my favorite." I love seeing the shocked and happy look on his face. Then I run to Henry's room and whisper the same thing to him before crawling back into my own bed.

There are even fewer studies of sleep and the siblings of neurodiverse kids than there are of parents! What research exists finds that about 20 percent of neurotypical siblings have a sleep problem directly related to their neurodiverse sibling.[9] This may be difficulty falling asleep or being woken at night, regardless of whether they share a room with their neurodiverse sibling or not.[10] Siblings of children with Down syndrome report minor sleep disruptions due to their sibling being awake, but major sleep disruptions from worry about their parents and sibling.

In my observation, neurotypical siblings have incredible amounts of empathy for others. They are tolerant and flexible of the normal variations in human beings. Neurotypical siblings try to help their neurodiverse sibling sleep better. They are more independent with their own routines and keep their sleep problems to themselves, believing they are normal and inevitable.[11] While they may be trying to help their parents, it also prevents parents from being able to help them. Neurotypical siblings often feel frustrated about having to stick to routines. Despite their frustration, they report understanding that their families have specific bedtime routines so that their neurodivergent sibling can have better sleep, and as a result, the whole family will have better sleep.

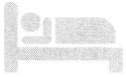

Tuck-In Tips

- A neurodiverse child's sleep problems can impact the mental and physical health of everyone in the family.
- If you're going to have even a sliver of a chance of living forever, self-care is critical.
- Ways to facilitate self-preservation include fostering community, religion or meditation, connecting with the present, interacting with living things, entertainment and/or distraction, maintaining routines, and managing overload.
- Keep an eye on the sleep of your neurotypical children, who tend to keep their sleep concerns and frustrations to themselves.

Pillow Point

Consider what helps the whole family sleep best, and don't forget your own self-care, whatever that may entail.

Epilogue

I wrote this epilogue the afternoon following my last DIY writing retreat. For the sixth and final time, I stayed in a hotel for the night to work on this book. As I was driving home, I felt a little wistful because, while this book has taken more work, time, and time away than I anticipated, I also loved writing it.

For the first time in twelve years, I let my mom and husband take over some of my responsibilities at home so that I could immerse myself in my writing. I thought about how I would probably miss the unique fulfillment that comes from being so fully engaged in a project that you forget yourself. Yet as I was driving and thinking all this, I could barely wait to get home to see my family. I ran inside and was reminded that Henry was at art camp and Simon was at a birthday party. I walked over to pick Henry up from camp. He ran out and gave me the biggest hug. He was a smidge teary as he told me how much he missed me, and he asked if I had finally finished my book.

"Mostly," I said.

"Does this mean you're going to be home more?" he asked. "Will you be with us more like you used to be?"

When I nodded, he pumped his fist in the air and gave a "YESSSSSS." He rode his scooter alongside me, and as we walked home, he said, "I guess my wish came true then. I've been wishing on a star that you would finish your book and be with me more."

I swallowed the lump in my throat and pulled him in for a hug, wondering, *What could ever be better than this?* as well as *Oh no, did I totally eff up my kids?*

Nothing unique about this. I know these simultaneous thoughts are pretty much universal to parenting, as we try to be the best we can for our kids.

When we got home, Simon was still at the birthday party, and Henry started working on a puzzle. It was the perfect time for Henry and me to have some quality togetherness and perhaps for me to smooth over any remaining sting from my nights away. I sat down on the floor beside him.

Before I even picked up one piece, he said, "Umm, Mommy? I want to do this by myself."

I acquiesced and told him that I just wanted to be near him. Less than a minute later, he sputtered, "Could you please…would you please…I need you to…please…Mommy, would you please go? I want some…I need some…I just want some time to be alone with my puzzle. I love you, and I want to be with you, but right now I need to be by myself with my puzzle so I can finish it."

I could feel his relief when I smiled and stood up to leave, understanding just how he felt.

Acknowledgments

Special thanks to the kind and exceptional people who have helped transform my dream book into reality: Chris Willard, for cheering me on before any words were written on the page; my agent, Linda Konner, for expert guidance and championing this book from day one; New World Library and my editor, Jason Gardner, for choosing this book, validating my ideas, and helping me create its best version; NWL Managing Editor Kristen Cashman and my copy editor, Jeff Campbell, whose editorial wizardry brought clarity, precision, and care to the finish line; Publicity Director Kim Corbin for enthusiastically ushering it into the world; my brother Dave, for the amazing website and design, and Sara, not only a sister-in-law but a wonderful colleague.

To the families who have been the core of my career, never-ending thank-yous.

Thank you to the incomparable Children's Hospital of Philadelphia Sleep Team for decades of brilliance, dedication, and laughter: Alex, Arun, Caitlin, Chris, Danna, Funke, Jeff, Jocelyn, Julie, Lee, Leo, Lourdes, Mary Kate, Melissa, Sue, Tina, Wendy; and all our outstanding trainees. Thanks to my new colleagues Rakesh and Eve, for being wonderful humans.

I would not be me without my mentors. I am forever grateful to Jodi Mindell, for endless time, opportunities, expertise, support, and friendship; to Carole Marcus, Denny Drotar, and Bob

Butler (all pioneers gone too soon), along with Terry Stancin, Lisa Meltzer, Sandra Russ, Norah Feeny, and Susan Redline, for wisdom and support along the way.

Love and thanks to my people:

- Our incredible Philly team, for their skill and support in helping us reach the surface and stay afloat: Susan Chaplick, Susan Hoban, Beth Boylan, Kiara Kendrick, Joelle McGovern, and Ali Downes
- David Santiago Speck, Chris Borkgren, and Ardiani Wang, along with PCDA, Ride-On, and ELARC — our California allies — who have helped us surpass our hopes for school and beyond
- Melissa and Anne, for showing me how it's done with intelligence and grace
- The inimitable Ignacio, for being the funniest, smartest, best colleague and friend
- Nadine and the Bayalas and the Dannemans, for being family
- The phenomenal friends who have lifted me up and laughed alongside me: Ariel, Courtney, Kathy, Victoria, Debra, Emily, Kristi, Terri, and Teresa
- Extra huge love to my Jenny for thirty years of unwavering friendship

Most importantly, colossal love and gratitude to my family:

- My kids, who are my raison d'être
- Charlie, the anchor who makes everything possible
- My mom, for enduring love, support, and erroneously believing I could do anything
- My dad, for a persistent belief in me and an unmatched sense of humor
- Brooke, Dave, and Matt, for giving me a lifelong sense of

belonging and the best nieces (Maren and June), nephews (Sutton, Beckett, Archer, and Cass), and in-laws (the Solomon family, Rebecca, and Eddie)

- Grandma and Jill, for always taking care of me
- The Shimeks (Michael, Stephen, Missy, and Stephanie), the Seymours (Charlie, Kate, Will, and Brian), the Bartkowskis (Christie and Eric), and the English fam (Bubber, Nubie, and Ann), for years of love, so much laughter, and hands all around

Endnotes

Chapter 1: In the Beginning

1. Karen A. Thomas, Robert L. Burr, and Susan Spieker, "Light and Maternal Influence in the Entrainment of Activity Circadian Rhythm in Infants 4–12 Weeks of Age," *Sleep and Biological Rhythms* 14, no. 3 (January 5, 2016): 249–55, https://doi.org/10.1007/s41105-015-0046-2; and Jacqueline M. Henderson et al., "Sleeping Through the Night: The Consolidation of Self-Regulated Sleep Across the First Year of Life," *Pediatrics* 126, no. 5 (November 1, 2010), https://doi.org/10.1542/peds.2010-0976.

2. Althea Robinson Shelton and Beth Malow, "Neurodevelopmental Disorders Commonly Presenting with Sleep Disturbances," *Neurotherapeutics* 18, no. 1 (January 2021): 156–69, https://doi.org/10.1007/s13311-020-00982-8; and Zaynab Mohamed et al., "Infant Sleep Characteristics in Children with Autism Spectrum Disorder: A Population-Derived Australian Birth Cohort Study," *Archives of Disease in Childhood* 110, no. 6 (May 11, 2025): 471–79, https://doi.org/10.1136/archdischild-2024-328393.

3. "Concerned About Your Child's Development?," Centers for Disease Control and Prevention, June 6, 2023, https://www.cdc.gov/act-early/families/concerned.html.

4. Shelton and Malow, "Neurodevelopmental Disorders Commonly Presenting."

5. E. Mark Mahone and Martha B. Denckla, "Attention-Deficit/Hyperactivity Disorder: A Historical Neuropsychological Perspective," *Journal of the International Neuropsychological Society* 23, no. 9–10 (October 2017): 916–29, https://doi.org/10.1017/s1355617717000807.

Chapter 3: What Is Healthy Sleep for Neurodiverse Kids

1. Shalini Paruthi et al., "Recommended Amount of Sleep for Pediatric Populations: A Consensus Statement of the American Academy of Sleep Medicine," *Journal of Clinical Sleep Medicine* 12, no. 6 (June 15, 2016): 785–86, https://doi.org/10.5664/jcsm.5866.

2. Mona El-Sheikh et al., "What Does a Good Night's Sleep Mean? Nonlinear Relations between Sleep and Children's Cognitive Functioning and Mental Health," *Sleep* 42, no. 6 (April 4, 2019), https://doi.org/10.1093/sleep/zsz078.
3. Daniel J. Buysse, "Sleep Health: Can We Define It? Does It Matter?," *Sleep* 37, no. 1 (January 1, 2014): 9–17, https://doi.org/10.5665/sleep.3298.
4. Lisa J. Meltzer, Ariel A. Williamson, and Jodi A. Mindell, "Pediatric Sleep Health: It Matters, and So Does How We Define It," *Sleep Medicine Reviews* 57 (June 2021): 101425, https://doi.org/10.1016/j.smrv.2021.101425.

Chapter 4: Why Do Neurodiverse Kids Have So Many Sleep Problems?

1. Terry Katz and Beth A. Malow, *Solving Sleep Problems in Children with Autism Spectrum Disorders: A Guide for Frazzled Families* (Woodbine House, 2014).
2. Angela Maxwell-Horn and Beth A. Malow, "Sleep in Autism," *Seminars in Neurology* 37, no. 4 (2017): 413–18; and Beth A. Malow et al., "Teaching Children with Autism Spectrum Disorder How to Sleep Better: A Pilot Educational Program for Parents," *Clinical Practice in Pediatric Psychology* 4, no. 2 (June 2016): 125–36, https://doi.org/10.1037/cpp0000138.
3. Sarika U. Peters et al., "A Clinical-Translational Review of Sleep Problems in Neurodevelopmental Disabilities," *Journal of Neurodevelopmental Disorders* 16, no. 1 (July 20, 2024), https://doi.org/10.1186/s11689-024-09559-4.
4. Beata Tick et al., "Heritability of Autism Spectrum Disorders: A Meta-analysis of Twin Studies," *Journal of Child Psychology and Psychiatry* 57, no. 5 (December 27, 2015): 585–95; and Stephen V. Faraone and Henrik Larsson, "Genetics of Attention Deficit Hyperactivity Disorder," *Molecular Psychiatry* 24, no. 4 (2018): 562–75.
5. Ayelet Arazi et al., "Reduced Sleep Pressure in Young Children with Autism," *Sleep* 43, no. 6 (December 18, 2019), https://doi.org/10.1093/sleep/zsz309.
6. Shelley A. Tischkau and Stacey L. Krager, "Orchestration of the Circadian Clock Network by the Suprachiasmatic Nucleus," *Neuronal Networks in Brain Function, CNS Disorders, and Therapeutics* (2014): 179–92, https://doi.org/10.1016/b978-0-12-415804-7.00014-9.
7. Wenjun Ding et al., "Research Progress on Melatonin, 5-HT, and Orexin in Sleep Disorders of Children with Autism Spectrum Disorder," *Biomolecules and Biomedicine* 25, no. 3 (January 30, 2025): 525–33, https://doi.org/10.17305/bb.2024.11182.
8. Ahmed Bouteldja et al., "The Circadian System: A Neglected Player in Neurodevelopmental Disorders," *European Journal of Neuroscience* 60, no. 2 (May 30, 2024): 3858–90, https://doi.org/10.1111/ejn.16423.
9. Jaclyn M. Kamradt, Allison M. Momany, and Molly A. Nikolas, "A Meta-Analytic Review of the Association Between Cortisol Reactivity in Response to a Stressor and Attention-Deficit Hyperactivity Disorder," *ADHD Attention Deficit and Hyperactivity Disorders* 10, no. 2 (September 5, 2017): 99–111, https://doi.org/10.1007/s12402-017-0238-5.

10. Scott A. Van Lenten and Leah D. Doane, "Examining Multiple Sleep Behaviors and Diurnal Salivary Cortisol and Alpha-Amylase: Within- and Between-Person Associations," *Psychoneuroendocrinology* 68 (June 2016): 100–110, https://doi.org/10.1016/j.psyneuen.2016.02.017; and Gerasimos Makris et al., "Stress System Activation in Children and Adolescents with Autism Spectrum Disorder," *Frontiers in Neuroscience* 15 (January 13, 2022), https://doi.org/10.3389/fnins.2021.756628.

11. Michael D. Greicius et al., "Functional Connectivity in the Resting Brain: A Network Analysis of the Default Mode Hypothesis," *Proceedings of the National Academy of Sciences* 100, no. 1 (December 27, 2002): 253–58, https://doi.org/10.1073/pnas.0135058100.

12. Silvina G. Horovitz et al., "Decoupling of the Brain's Default Mode Network During Deep Sleep," *Proceedings of the National Academy of Sciences* 106, no. 27 (July 7, 2009): 11376–81, https://doi.org/10.1073/pnas.0901435106.

13. A. C. Linke et al., "Sleep Problems in Preschoolers with Autism Spectrum Disorders Are Associated with Sensory Sensitivities and Thalamocortical Overconnectivity," *Biological Psychiatry: Cognitive Neuroscience and Neuroimaging* (January 15, 2021), https://doi.org/10.1101/2021.01.15.426899.

14. Nadia Aalling Jessen et al., "The Glymphatic System: A Beginner's Guide," *Neurochemical Research* 40, no. 12 (May 7, 2015): 2583–99, https://doi.org/10.1007/s11064-015-1581-6.

15. Yingqian Chen et al., "Assessment of the Glymphatic Function in Children with Attention-Deficit/Hyperactivity Disorder," *European Radiology* 34, no. 3 (September 6, 2023): 1444–52, https://doi.org/10.1007/s00330-023-10220-2; Dea Garic et al., "Enlarged Perivascular Spaces in Infancy and Autism Diagnosis, Cerebrospinal Fluid Volume, and Later Sleep Problems," *JAMA Network Open* 6, no. 12 (December 19, 2023), https://doi.org/10.1001/jamanetworkopen.2023.48341; and Ruifang Xiong et al., "Evaluation of Glymphatic System Dysfunction in Patients with Insomnia via Diffusion Tensor Image Analysis Along the Perivascular Space," *Quantitative Imaging in Medicine and Surgery* 15, no. 2 (February 2025): 1114–24, https://doi.org/10.21037/qims-24-1447.

16. Shelton and Malow, "Neurodevelopmental Disorders Commonly Presenting" (see chap. 1, n. 2); and Zaynab Mohamed et al., "Infant Sleep Characteristics in Children with Autism Spectrum Disorder: A Population-Derived Australian Birth Cohort Study," *Archives of Disease in Childhood* 110, no. 6 (May 11, 2025): 471–79, https://doi.org/10.1136/archdischild-2024-328393.

Chapter 5: Is It a Medical Sleep Disorder?

1. Ron B. Mitchell et al., "Clinical Characteristics of Primary Snoring vs Mild Obstructive Sleep Apnea in Children," *JAMA Otolaryngology–Head & Neck Surgery* 150, no. 2 (February 1, 2024): 99, https://doi.org/10.1001/jamaoto.2023.3816.

2. E. I. Verhelst et al., "Positional Obstructive Sleep Apnea in Children: Prevalence and Risk Factors," *Sleep and Breathing* 23, no. 4 (May 7, 2019): 1323–30, https://doi.org/10.1007/s11325-019-01853-z.

3. Carole L. Marcus et al., "A Randomized Trial of Adenotonsillectomy for Childhood Sleep Apnea," *New England Journal of Medicine* 368, no. 25 (June 20, 2013): 2366–76, https://doi.org/10.1056/nejmoa1215881.

4. Joel Reiter, "Treatment of OSA Beyond Adenotonsillectomy," *Pediatric Pulmonology* 60, no. S1 (October 22, 2024), https://doi.org/10.1002/ppul.27297.

5. Melissa S. Xanthopoulos et al., "Caregiver Experiences Helping Children with Down Syndrome Use Positive Airway Pressure to Treat Obstructive Sleep Apnea," *Sleep Medicine* 107 (July 2023): 179–86, https://doi.org/10.1016/j.sleep.2023.04.022.

6. Mandeep Rana et al., "Alternative Approaches to Adenotonsillectomy and Continuous Positive Airway Pressure (CPAP) for the Management of Pediatric Obstructive Sleep Apnea (OSA): A Review," *Sleep Disorders* 2020 (July 4, 2020): 1–11, https://doi.org/10.1155/2020/7987208.

7. Chun Ting Au et al., "Sleep Apnea-Specific Hypoxic Burden and Pulse Rate Response in Children Using High Flow Nasal Cannula Therapy Compared with Continuous Positive Airway Pressure," *Sleep Medicine* 124 (December 2024): 187–90, https://doi.org/10.1016/j.sleep.2024.09.032.

8. Ignacio E. Tapia et al., "A Trial of Intranasal Corticosteroids to Treat Childhood OSA Syndrome," *Chest* 162, no. 4 (October 2022): 899–919, https://doi.org/10.1016/j.chest.2022.06.026.

9. Michael G. Aman et al., "A Review of Atomoxetine Effects in Young People with Developmental Disabilities," *Research in Developmental Disabilities* 35, no. 6 (June 2014): 1412–24, https://doi.org/10.1016/j.ridd.2014.03.006; and Daniel Combs et al., "The Combination of Atomoxetine and Oxybutynin for the Treatment of Obstructive Sleep Apnea in Children with Down Syndrome," *Journal of Clinical Sleep Medicine* 19, no. 12 (December 2023): 2065–73, https://doi.org/10.5664/jcsm.10764.

10. Michael W. Noller et al., "Mandibular Advancement for Pediatric Obstructive Sleep Apnea: A Systematic Review and Meta-Analysis," *Journal of Cranio-Maxillofacial Surgery* 46, no. 8 (August 2018): 1296–1302, https://doi.org/10.1016/j.jcms.2018.04.027; Clete A. Kushida et al., "Multicenter Clinical Trial for the Treatment of Obstructive Sleep Apnea with a Non-Permanent Orthodontic Intraoral Device in Children," *European Journal of Pediatrics* 184, no. 7 (June 17, 2025), https://doi.org/10.1007/s00431-025-06254-x; and Macario Camacho et al., "Rapid Maxillary Expansion for Pediatric Obstructive Sleep Apnea: A Systematic Review and Meta-Analysis," *The Laryngoscope* 127, no. 7 (October 31, 2016): 1712–19, https://doi.org/10.1002/lary.26352.

11. Macario Camacho et al., "Tongue Surgeries for Pediatric Obstructive Sleep Apnea: A Systematic Review and Meta-Analysis," *European Archives of Oto-Rhino-Laryngology* 274, no. 8 (April 4, 2017): 2981–90, https://doi.org/10.1007/s00405-017-4545-4.

12. Maoyu Ye et al., "The Therapeutic Role of Orofacial Myofunctional Therapy in Childhood Residual Obstructive Sleep Apnea," *Pediatric Pulmonology* 60, no. 2 (February 2025), https://doi.org/10.1002/ppul.70993.

13. Claudia de Felicio, Franciele Dias, and Luciana Trawitzki, "Obstructive Sleep Apnea: Focus on Myofunctional Therapy," *Nature and Science of Sleep* 10 (September 2018): 271–86, https://doi.org/10.2147/nss.s141132.

14. Jurjen C. de Jong et al., "The Impact of Playing a Musical Instrument on Obstructive Sleep Apnea: A Systematic Review," *Annals of Otology, Rhinology & Laryngology* 129, no. 9 (May 4, 2020): 924–29, https://doi.org/10.1177/0003489420917407.

15. Oliviero Bruni et al., "L-5-Hydroxytryptophan Treatment of Sleep Terrors in Children," *European Journal of Pediatrics* 163, no. 7 (May 14, 2004), https://doi.org/10.1007/s00431-004-1444-7; and Louis T. van Zyl et al., "L-Tryptophan as Treatment for Pediatric Non-Rapid Eye Movement Parasomnia," *Journal of Child and Adolescent Psychopharmacology* 28, no. 6 (August 2018): 395–401, https://doi.org/10.1089/cap.2017.0164.

16. Elisa Pellegrini et al., "Behind Closed Eyes: Understanding Nightmares in Children and Adolescents with Autism Spectrum Disorder — A Systematic Review," *Neuroscience & Biobehavioral Reviews* 169 (February 2025): 106012, https://doi.org/10.1016/j.neubiorev.2025.106012.

17. Peter Gill et al., "Psychosocial Treatments for Nightmares in Adults and Children: A Systematic Review," *BMC Psychiatry* 23, no. 1 (April 21, 2023), https://doi.org/10.1186/s12888-023-04703-1.

18. Lisa DeMarni Cromer, Brooke A. Pangelinan, and Tara R. Buck, "Case Study of Cognitive Behavioral Therapy for Nightmares in Children With and Without Trauma History," *Clinical Case Studies* 21, no. 5 (April 4, 2022): 377–95, https://doi.org/10.1177/15346501221081122; and Lisa DeMarni Cromer et al., "Efficacy of a Telehealth Cognitive Behavioral Therapy for Improving Sleep and Nightmares in Children Aged 6–17," *Frontiers in Sleep* 3 (July 11, 2024), https://doi.org/10.3389/frsle.2024.1401023.

19. Daniel L. Picchietti et al., "Pediatric Restless Legs Syndrome: Analysis of Symptom Descriptions and Drawings," *Journal of Child Neurology* 26, no. 11 (June 2, 2011): 1365–76, https://doi.org/10.1177/0883073811405852.

20. Sharon Tamir, Thomas J. Dye, and Rochelle M. Witt, "Sleep and Circadian Disturbances in Children with Neurodevelopmental Disorders," *Seminars in Pediatric Neurology* 48 (December 2023): 101090, https://doi.org/10.1016/j.spen.2023.101090.

21. Stephanie J. Crowley, Christine Acebo, and Mary A. Carskadon, "Sleep, Circadian Rhythms, and Delayed Phase in Adolescence," *Sleep Medicine* 8, no. 6 (September 2007): 602–12, https://doi.org/10.1016/j.sleep.2006.12.002.

22. R. Robert Auger et al., "Clinical Practice Guideline for the Treatment of Intrinsic Circadian Rhythm Sleep-Wake Disorders: Advanced Sleep-Wake Phase Disorder (ASWPD), Delayed Sleep-Wake Phase Disorder (DSWPD), Non-24-Hour Sleep-Wake Rhythm Disorder (N24SWD), and

Irregular Sleep-Wake Rhythm Disorder (ISWRD): An Update for 2015," *Journal of Clinical Sleep Medicine* 11, no. 10 (October 15, 2015): 1199–1236, https://doi.org/10.5664/jcsm.5100.

23. N. Hajjaj and D. Henry, "Kleine-Levin Syndrome: A Clinical Challenge in Pediatric Hypersomnia," *American Journal of Respiratory and Critical Care Medicine* 211, no. Abstracts (May 2025), https://doi.org/10.1164/ajrccm.2025.211.abstracts.a7857.

Chapter 6: What If It's Not a Medical Sleep Disorder?

1. A. Spielman, "Assessment of Insomnia," *Clinical Psychology Review* 6, no. 1 (1986): 11–25, https://doi.org/10.1016/0272-7358(86)90015-2; Juan J. Madrid-Valero, Nicola L. Barclay, and Alice M. Gregory, "The Interaction between Polygenic Risk and Environmental Influences: A Direct Test of the 3P Model of Insomnia in Adolescents," *Journal of Child Psychology and Psychiatry* 65, no. 3 (October 4, 2023): 308–15, https://doi.org/10.1111/jcpp.13895; Noller et al., "Mandibular Advancement for Pediatric" (chap. 5, n. 10); and Julia Dewald-Kaufmann, Ed de Bruin, and Gradisar Michael, "Cognitive Behavioral Therapy for Insomnia (CBT-i) in School-Aged Children and Adolescents," *Sleep Medicine Clinics* 14, no. 2 (June 2019): 155–65, https://doi.org/10.1016/j.jsmc.2019.02.002.

Chapter 7: What If the Sleep Problem Isn't Caused by a Sleep Disorder?

1. Caspar Bundgaard-Nielsen et al., "Gut Microbiota Profiles of Autism Spectrum Disorder and Attention Deficit/Hyperactivity Disorder: A Systematic Literature Review," *Gut Microbes* 11, no. 5 (April 24, 2020): 1172–87, https://doi.org/10.1080/19490976.2020.1748258.

2. Petra Zimmermann et al., "Association Between the Intestinal Microbiota and Allergic Sensitization, Eczema, and Asthma: A Systematic Review," *Journal of Allergy and Clinical Immunology* 143, no. 2 (February 2019): 467–85, https://doi.org/10.1016/j.jaci.2018.09.025.

3. Regena Xin Chua et al., "Understanding the Link Between Allergy and Neurodevelopmental Disorders: A Current Review of Factors and Mechanisms," *Frontiers in Neurology* 11 (February 15, 2021), https://doi.org/10.3389/fneur.2020.603571.

4. Mairav Cohen-Zion and Sonia Ancoli-Israel, "Sleep in Children with Attention-Deficit Hyperactivity Disorder (ADHD): A Review of Naturalistic and Stimulant Intervention Studies," *Sleep Medicine Reviews* 8, no. 5 (October 2004): 379–402, https://doi.org/10.1016/j.smrv.2004.06.002.

5. Connor M. Kerns et al., "Clinically Significant Anxiety in Children with Autism Spectrum Disorder and Varied Intellectual Functioning," *Journal of Clinical Child & Adolescent Psychology* 50, no. 6 (January 23, 2020): 780–95, https://doi.org/10.1080/15374416.2019.1703712; and Emma

Sciberras et al., "Anxiety in Children with Attention-Deficit/Hyperactivity Disorder," *Pediatrics* 133, no. 5 (May 1, 2014): 801–8, https://doi.org /10.1542/peds.2013-3686.

6. Pasquale K. Alvaro et al., "The Direction of the Relationship Between Symptoms of Insomnia and Psychiatric Disorders in Adolescents," *Journal of Affective Disorders* 207 (January 2017): 167–74, https://doi.org/10.1016 /j.jad.2016.08.032.

7. Olga Eyre et al., "Childhood Neurodevelopmental Difficulties and Risk of Adolescent Depression: The Role of Irritability," *Journal of Child Psychology and Psychiatry* 60, no. 8 (March 25, 2019): 866–74, https://doi.org /10.1111/jcpp.13053.

8. Danielle Ung et al., "A Systematic Review and Meta-Analysis of Cognitive-Behavioral Therapy for Anxiety in Youth with High-Functioning Autism Spectrum Disorders," *Child Psychiatry & Human Development* 46, no. 4 (September 23, 2014): 533–47, https://doi.org/10.1007/s10578-014 -0494-y.

9. Camille Hours, Christophe Recasens, and Jean-Marc Baleyte, "ASD and ADHD Comorbidity: What Are We Talking About?," *Frontiers in Psychiatry* 13 (February 28, 2022), https://doi.org/10.3389/fpsyt.2022.837424.

10. Jianghong Liu et al., "The Bidirectional Relationship Between Sleep and Externalizing Behavior: A Systematic Review," *Sleep Epidemiology* 2 (December 2022): 100039, https://doi.org/10.1016/j.sleepe.2022.100039.

11. Claire Whiting et al., "Associations Between Sleep Quality and Irritability: Testing the Mediating Role of Emotion Regulation," *Personality and Individual Differences* 213 (October 2023), https://doi.org/10.2139/ssrn.4386988.

Chapter 8: Does This Stuff Apply to Children with Rare Conditions?

1. Linda Horwood et al., "A Systematic Review and Meta-Analysis of the Prevalence of Sleep Problems in Children with Cerebral Palsy: How Do Children with Cerebral Palsy Differ from Each Other and from Typically Developing Children?," *Sleep Health* 5, no. 6 (December 2019): 555–71, https://doi.org/10.1016/j.sleh.2019.08.006; Katarzyna Anna Dylag et al., "Sleep Problems Among Children with Fetal Alcohol Spectrum Disorders (FASD) — An Explorative Study," *Italian Journal of Pediatrics* 47, no. 1 (May 17, 2021), https://doi.org/10.1186/s13052-021-01056-x; and Dagmara Annaz et al., "Characterisation of Sleep Problems in Children with Williams Syndrome," *Research in Developmental Disabilities* 32, no. 1 (January 2011): 164–69, https://doi.org/10.1016/j.ridd.2010.09.008.

Chapter 10: Communicate About Sleep

1. Carol A. Gray and Joy D. Garand, "Social Stories: Improving Responses of Students with Autism with Accurate Social Information," *Focus on Autistic Behavior* 8, no. 1 (April 1993): 1–10, https://doi.org/10.1177/108835769 300800101.

Chapter 11: Open the Door for Sleep
(aka the Dreaded Sleep Hygiene)

1. Jodi A. Mindell and Ariel A. Williamson, "Benefits of a Bedtime Routine in Young Children: Sleep, Development, and Beyond," *Sleep Medicine Reviews* 40 (August 2018): 93–108, https://doi.org/10.1016/j.smrv.2017.10.007; and Jodi A. Mindell et al., "Bedtime Routines for Young Children: A Dose-Dependent Association with Sleep Outcomes," *Sleep* 38, no. 5 (May 1, 2015): 717–22, https://doi.org/10.5665/sleep.4662.
2. Mindell et al., "Bedtime Routines for Young Children."
3. Christian Cajochen et al., "Evening Exposure to a Light-Emitting Diodes (LED)-Backlit Computer Screen Affects Circadian Physiology and Cognitive Performance," *Journal of Applied Physiology* 110, no. 5 (May 2011): 1432–38, https://doi.org/10.1152/japplphysiol.00165.2011.
4. Judith Owens et al., "Television-Viewing Habits and Sleep Disturbance in School Children," *Pediatrics* 104, no. 3 (September 1, 1999), https://doi.org/10.1542/peds.104.3.e27.
5. Serena Bauducco et al., "A Bidirectional Model of Sleep and Technology Use: A Theoretical Review of How Much, for Whom, and Which Mechanisms," *Sleep Medicine Reviews* 76 (August 2024): 101933, https://doi.org/10.1016/j.smrv.2024.101933.
6. Ben Hinnant et al., "Socioeconomic Disparities, Nighttime Bedroom Temperature, and Children's Sleep," *Journal of Applied Developmental Psychology* 86 (May 2023): 101530, https://doi.org/10.1016/j.appdev.2023.101530.
7. Shahab Haghayegh et al., "Before-Bedtime Passive Body Heating by Warm Shower or Bath to Improve Sleep: A Systematic Review and Meta-Analysis," *Sleep Medicine Reviews* 46 (August 2019): 124–35, https://doi.org/10.1016/j.smrv.2019.04.008.

Chapter 12: Waiting for Sleep to Arrive

1. L. Beaudoin et al., "Towards an Integrative Design-Oriented Theory of Sleep-Onset and Insomnolence from Which a New Cognitive Treatment for Insomnolence (Serial Diverse Kinesthetic Imagining, a Form of Cognitive Shuffling) Is Proposed for Experimentally Testing This Against Alternatives," *Sleep Medicine* 64 (December 2019), https://doi.org/10.1016/j.sleep.2019.11.081.

Chapter 13: Bedtime Conflicts and Positive Sleep Associations

1. B. A. Moore et al., "Brief Report: Evaluating the Bedtime Pass Program for Child Resistance to Bedtime — A Randomized, Controlled Trial," *Journal of Pediatric Psychology* 32, no. 3 (June 23, 2006): 283–87, https://doi.org/10.1093/jpepsy/jsl025.

Chapter 15: Nighttime Fears, Worries, and Distressing Thoughts

1. Peter Muris et al., "Children's Nighttime Fears: Parent–Child Ratings of Frequency, Content, Origins, Coping Behaviors and Severity," *Behaviour Research and Therapy* 39, no. 1 (January 2001): 13–28, https:// doi.org/10.1016/s0005-7967(99)00155-2; and Jocelynne Gordon et al., "Nighttime Fears of Children and Adolescents: Frequency, Content, Severity, Harm Expectations, Disclosure, and Coping Behaviours," *Behaviour Research and Therapy* 45, no. 10 (October 2007): 2464–72, https://doi .org/10.1016/j.brat.2007.03.013.
2. Jonathan Kushnir and Avi Sadeh, "Assessment of Brief Interventions for Nighttime Fears in Preschool Children," *European Journal of Pediatrics* 171, no. 1 (May 19, 2011): 67–75, https://doi.org/10.1007/s00431-011 -1488-4.

Chapter 16: Sensory Sensitivities and Stims

1. Molly Shields Bagby, Virginia A. Dickie, and Grace T. Baranek, "How Sensory Experiences of Children With and Without Autism Affect Family Occupations," *The American Journal of Occupational Therapy* 66, no. 1 (January 1, 2012): 78–86, https://doi.org/10.5014/ajot.2012.000604.
2. Liora Manelis-Baram et al., "Sleep Disturbances and Sensory Sensitivities Co-Vary in a Longitudinal Manner in Pre-School Children with Autism Spectrum Disorders," *Journal of Autism and Developmental Disorders* 52, no. 2 (April 9, 2021): 923–37, https://doi.org/10.1007/s10803-021-04973-2.
3. Amy S. Weitlauf et al., "Interventions Targeting Sensory Challenges in Autism Spectrum Disorder: A Systematic Review," *Pediatrics* 139, no. 6 (June 1, 2017), https://doi.org/10.1542/peds.2017-0347; and Jane Case-Smith, Lindy L. Weaver, and Mary A Fristad, "A Systematic Review of Sensory Processing Interventions for Children with Autism Spectrum Disorders," *Autism* 19, no. 2 (January 29, 2014): 133–48, https://doi.org /10.1177/1362361313517762.
4. Stephen Stansfeld and Charlotte Clark, "Health Effects of Noise Exposure in Children," *Current Environmental Health Reports* 2, no. 2 (March 26, 2015): 171–78, https://doi.org/10.1007/s40572-015-0044-1.
5. Samantha M. Riedy et al., "Noise as a Sleep Aid: A Systematic Review," *Sleep Medicine Reviews* 55 (February 2021): 101385, https://doi .org/10.1016/j.smrv.2020.101385; and Russell W. De Jong et al., "Continuous White Noise Exposure During Sleep and Childhood Development: A Scoping Review," *Sleep Medicine* 119 (July 2024): 88–94, https://doi .org/10.1016/j.sleep.2024.04.006.
6. Laura-Lee Kathleen McLay and Karyn France, "Empirical Research Evaluating Non-Traditional Approaches to Managing Sleep Problems in Children with Autism," *Developmental Neurorehabilitation* (April 11, 2014): 1–12, https://doi.org/10.3109/17518423.2014.904452.
7. Suzanne Dawson et al., "Weighted Blankets as a Sleep Intervention: A

Scoping Review," *The American Journal of Occupational Therapy* 78, no. 5 (August 20, 2024), https://doi.org/10.5014/ajot.2024.050676.

8. Georgia Pavlopoulou, "A Good Night's Sleep: Learning About Sleep from Autistic Adolescents' Personal Accounts," *Frontiers in Psychology* 11 (December 22, 2020), https://doi.org/10.3389/fpsyg.2020.583868.

9. Maria Clince, Laura Connolly, and Clodagh Nolan, "Comparing and Exploring the Sensory Processing Patterns of Higher Education Students with Attention Deficit Hyperactivity Disorder and Autism Spectrum Disorder," *The American Journal of Occupational Therapy* 70, no. 2 (January 14, 2016), https://doi.org/10.5014/ajot.2016.016816.

Chapter 17: Movement and Mindfulness

1. Christina F. Chick et al., "A School-Based Health and Mindfulness Curriculum Improves Children's Objectively Measured Sleep: A Prospective Observational Cohort Study," *Journal of Clinical Sleep Medicine* 18, no. 9 (September 2022): 2261–71, https://doi.org/10.5664/jcsm.9508.

2. Kristie Patten Koenig, Anne Buckley-Reen, and Satvika Garg, "Efficacy of the Get Ready to Learn Yoga Program Among Children with Autism Spectrum Disorders: A Pretest–Posttest Control Group Design," *The American Journal of Occupational Therapy* 66, no. 5 (September 1, 2012): 538–46, https://doi.org/10.5014/ajot.2012.004390.

3. YanAn Wang et al., "The Impact of Physical and Motor Skills in Children with Autism: A Systematic Review and Meta-Analysis of Randomized Exercise Interventions on Social, Behavioral, Controlled Trials" (January 14, 2025), https://doi.org/10.37766/inplasy2025.1.0046.

4. Andy C. Y. Tse et al., "Effects of Exercise on Sleep, Melatonin Level, and Behavioral Functioning in Children with Autism," *Autism* 26, no. 7 (January 27, 2022): 1712–22, https://doi.org/10.1177/13623613211062952.

5. Yoon-Suk Hwang and Patrick Kearney, "A Systematic Review of Mindfulness Intervention for Individuals with Developmental Disabilities: Long-Term Practice and Long-Lasting Effects," *Research in Developmental Disabilities* 34, no. 1 (January 2013): 314–26, https://doi.org/10.1016/j.ridd.2012.08.008; Anna Ridderinkhof et al., "Attention in Children with Autism Spectrum Disorder and the Effects of a Mindfulness-Based Program," *Journal of Attention Disorders* 24, no. 5 (September 15, 2018): 681–92, https://doi.org/10.1177/1087054718797428; and Vittoria Zaccari et al., "Clinical Application of Mindfulness-Oriented Meditation in Children with ADHD: A Preliminary Study on Sleep and Behavioral Problems," *Psychology & Health* (March 7, 2021): 1–17, https://doi.org/10.1080/08870446.2021.1892110.

6. Anna Ridderinkhof et al., "Mindfulness-Based Program for Autism Spectrum Disorder: A Qualitative Study of the Experiences of Children and Parents," *Mindfulness* 10, no. 9 (July 16, 2019): 1936–51, https://doi.org/10.1007/s12671-019-01202-x.

7. Pavlopoulou, "Good Night's Sleep" (chap. 16, n. 8).

Chapter 18: Melatonin, Magnesium, Marijuana, and Medications

1. P. Gail Williams, Lonnie L. Sears, and AnnaMary Allard, "Sleep Problems in Children with Autism," *Journal of Sleep Research* 13, no. 3 (September 2004): 265–68, https://doi.org/10.1111/j.1365-2869.2004.00405.x.

2. Junaura Rocha Barretto, Mara Alves Gouveia, and Crésio Alves, "Use of Dietary Supplements by Children and Adolescents," *Jornal de Pediatria* 100 (March 2024), https://doi.org/10.1016/j.jped.2023.09.008; and Anita A. Panjwani et al., "Trends in Nutrient- and Non-Nutrient–Containing Dietary Supplement Use Among US Children from 1999 to 2016," *The Journal of Pediatrics* 231 (April 2021), https://doi.org/10.1016/j.jpeds.2020.12.021.

3. "FDA 101: Dietary Supplements," US Food and Drug Administration, Office of the Commissioner, accessed July 17, 2025, https://www.fda.gov/consumers/consumer-updates/fda-101-dietary-supplements.

4. Pieter A. Cohen et al., "Quantity of Melatonin and CBD in Melatonin Gummies Sold in the US," *JAMA* 329, no. 16 (April 25, 2023): 1401, https://doi.org/10.1001/jama.2023.2296; and Lauren A. E. Erland and Praveen K. Saxena, "Melatonin Natural Health Products and Supplements: Presence of Serotonin and Significant Variability of Melatonin Content," *Journal of Clinical Sleep Medicine* 13, no. 2 (February 15, 2017): 275–81, https://doi.org/10.5664/jcsm.6462.

5. R. E. Appleton et al., "The Use of Melatonin in Children with Neurodevelopmental Disorders and Impaired Sleep: A Randomised, Double-Blind, Placebo-Controlled, Parallel Study (MENDS)," *Health Technology Assessment* 16, no. 40 (October 2012), https://doi.org/10.3310/hta16400.

6. Lisa M. Bendz and Ann C. Scates, "Melatonin Treatment for Insomnia in Pediatric Patients with Attention-Deficit/Hyperactivity Disorder," *Annals of Pharmacotherapy* 44, no. 1 (January 2010): 185–91, https://doi.org/10.1345/aph.1m365.

7. Michel Hoebert et al., "Long-Term Follow-Up of Melatonin Treatment in Children with ADHD and Chronic Sleep Onset Insomnia," *Journal of Pineal Research* 47, no. 1 (July 2009): 1–7, https://doi.org/10.1111/j.1600-079x.2009.00681.x.

8. Beth A. Malow et al., "Sleep, Growth, and Puberty After 2 Years of Prolonged-Release Melatonin in Children with Autism Spectrum Disorder," *Journal of the American Academy of Child & Adolescent Psychiatry* 60, no. 2 (February 2021), https://doi.org/10.1016/j.jaac.2019.12.007.

9. Nave Zisapel, "Assessing the Potential for Drug Interactions and Long Term Safety of Melatonin for the Treatment of Insomnia in Children with Autism Spectrum Disorder," *Expert Review of Clinical Pharmacology* 15, no. 2 (February 1, 2022): 175–85, https://doi.org/10.1080/17512433.2022.2053520.

10. N. Buscemi et al., "Melatonin for Treatment of Sleep Disorders: Summary," National Library of Medicine, Agency for Healthcare Research and Quality Evidence Report Summaries, accessed July 17, 2025, https://www.ncbi.nlm.nih.gov/books/NBK11941.

11. Frank M. Besag and Michael J. Vasey, "Adverse Events in Long-Term Studies of Exogenous Melatonin," *Expert Opinion on Drug Safety* 21, no. 12 (December 2, 2022): 1469–81, https://doi.org/10.1080/14740338.2022.2160444.

12. P. Gringras et al., "Melatonin for Sleep Problems in Children with Neuro-developmental Disorders: Randomised Double Masked Placebo Controlled Trial," *BMJ* 345 (November 5, 2012), https://doi.org/10.1136/bmj.e6664.

13. Cyrille Feybesse, Sylvie Chokron, and Sylvie Tordjman, "Melatonin in Neurodevelopmental Disorders: A Critical Literature Review," *Antioxidants* 12, no. 11 (November 20, 2023): 2017, https://doi.org/10.3390/antiox12112017.

14. Olakunle J. Onaolapo and Adejoke Y. Onaolapo, "Melatonin in Drug Addiction and Addiction Management: Exploring an Evolving Multidimensional Relationship," *World Journal of Psychiatry* 8, no. 2 (June 28, 2018): 64–74, https://doi.org/10.5498/wjp.v8.i2.64.

15. J. A. Boutin, D. J. Kennaway, and R. Jockers, "Melatonin: Facts, Extrapolations, and Clinical Trials," *Biomolecules* 13, no. 6 (June 5, 2023): 943, https://doi.org/10.3390/biom13060943; and Yulin Sun et al., "Safety and Efficacy of Melatonin Supplementation as an Add-on Treatment for Infantile Epileptic Spasms Syndrome: A Randomized, Placebo-Controlled, Double-Blind Trial," *Journal of Pineal Research* 76, no. 1 (November 2023), https://doi.org/10.1111/jpi.12922.

16. Pranita Shenoy et al., "Melatonin Use in Pediatrics: A Clinical Review on Indications, Multisystem Effects, and Toxicity," *Children* 11, no. 3 (March 9, 2024): 323, https://doi.org/10.3390/children11030323.

17. Samuele Cortese et al., "Sleep Disturbances and Serum Ferritin Levels in Children with Attention-Deficit/Hyperactivity Disorder," *European Child & Adolescent Psychiatry* 18, no. 7 (February 5, 2009): 393–99, https://doi.org/10.1007/s00787-009-0746-8; and Maha K. Abou-Khadra et al., "Parent-Reported Sleep Problems, Symptom Ratings, and Serum Ferritin Levels in Children with Attention-Deficit/Hyperactivity Disorder: A Case Control Study," *BMC Pediatrics* 13, no. 1 (December 2013), https://doi.org/10.1186/1471-2431-13-217.

18. Kumars Pourrostami et al., "The Association Between Vitamin D Status and Sleep Duration in School-Aged Children: The CASPIAN-V Study," *Journal of Diabetes & Metabolic Disorders* 22, no. 1 (November 17, 2022): 341–46, https://doi.org/10.1007/s40200-022-01146-5.

19. Baha Al-Shawwa, Zarmina Ehsan, and David G. Ingram, "Vitamin D and Sleep in Children," *Journal of Clinical Sleep Medicine* 16, no. 7 (July 15, 2020): 1119–23, https://doi.org/10.5664/jcsm.8440.

20. Leila Kheirandish-Gozal, Eduard Peris, and David Gozal, "Vitamin D Levels and Obstructive Sleep Apnoea in Children," *Sleep Medicine* 15, no. 4 (April 2014): 459–63, https://doi.org/10.1016/j.sleep.2013.12.009; and Andrew E. Bluher et al., "Vitamin D Deficiency and Pediatric Obstructive Sleep Apnea Severity," *JAMA Otolaryngology–Head & Neck Surgery* 151,

no. 1 (January 1, 2025): 72, https://doi.org/10.1001/jamaoto.2024.3737.

21. Mohammad Effatpanah et al., "Magnesium Status and Attention Deficit Hyperactivity Disorder (ADHD): A Meta-Analysis," *Psychiatry Research* 274 (April 2019): 228–34, https://doi.org/10.1016/j.psychres.2019.02.043.

22. Mostafa Hemamy et al., "The Effect of Vitamin D and Magnesium Supplementation on the Mental Health Status of Attention-Deficit Hyperactive Children: A Randomized Controlled Trial," *BMC Pediatrics* 21, no. 1 (2021): 178, https://doi.org/10.1186/s12887-021-02631-1.

23. Ali Jadidi et al., "Therapeutic Effects of Magnesium and Vitamin B6 in Alleviating the Symptoms of Restless Legs Syndrome: A Randomized Controlled Clinical Trial," *BMC Complementary Medicine and Therapies* 23, no. 1 (December 31, 2022), https://doi.org/10.1186/s12906-022-03814-8.

24. James Adams et al., "Comprehensive Nutritional and Dietary Intervention for Autism Spectrum Disorder — A Randomized, Controlled 12-Month Trial," *Nutrients* 10, no. 3 (March 17, 2018): 369, https://doi.org/10.3390/nu10030369.

25. Bruni et al., "L-5-Hydroxytryptophan Treatment" (chap. 5, n. 15); and Zyl et al., "L-Tryptophan as Treatment for Pediatric" (chap. 5, n. 15).

26. Miyo Nakade et al., "Can Breakfast Tryptophan and Vitamin B6 Intake and Morning Exposure to Sunlight Promote Morning-Typology in Young Children Aged 2 to 6 Years?," *Journal of Physiological Anthropology* 31, no. 1 (May 22, 2012), https://doi.org/10.1186/1880-6805-31-11.

27. Mahmood AminiLari et al., "Medical Cannabis and Cannabinoids for Impaired Sleep: A Systematic Review and Meta-Analysis of Randomized Clinical Trials," *Sleep* 45, no. 2 (September 21, 2021), https://doi.org/10.1093/sleep/zsab234.

28. Danilo A. Pereira et al., "Efficacy and Safety of Cannabinoids for Autism Spectrum Disorder: An Updated Systematic Review," *Cureus*, March 17, 2025, https://doi.org/10.7759/cureus.80725; Estácio Amaro Silva Junior et al., "Cannabis and Cannabinoid Use in Autism Spectrum Disorder: A Systematic Review," *Trends in Psychiatry and Psychotherapy*, 2021, https://doi.org/10.47626/2237-6089-2020-0149; Adi Aran et al., "Brief Report: Cannabidiol-Rich Cannabis in Children with Autism Spectrum Disorder and Severe Behavioral Problems — A Retrospective Feasibility Study," *Journal of Autism and Developmental Disorders* 49, no. 3 (October 31, 2018): 1284–88, https://doi.org/10.1007/s10803-018-3808-2; and Dana Barchel et al., "Oral Cannabidiol Use in Children with Autism Spectrum Disorder to Treat Related Symptoms and Co-Morbidities," *Frontiers in Pharmacology* 9 (January 9, 2019), https://doi.org/10.3389/fphar.2018.01521.

29. Oliviero Bruni et al., "Practitioner Review: Treatment of Chronic Insomnia in Children and Adolescents with Neurodevelopmental Disabilities," *Journal of Child Psychology and Psychiatry* 59, no. 5 (September 18, 2017): 489–508, https://doi.org/10.1111/jcpp.12812; and Jessica Edwards, "Prescribing in the Dark: Off-Label Drug Treatments for Children with Insomnia," Association for Child and Adolescent Mental Health, December 20, 2023, https://www.acamh.org/research-digest

/prescribing-in-the-dark-off-label-drug-treatments-for-children-with
-insomnia.

30. Rahime Duygu Temeltürk et al., "Use of Clonidine in Attention Deficit
Hyperactivity Disorder and Autism Spectrum Disorder Comorbidity:
Report of 3 Cases," *Psychiatry and Clinical Psychopharmacology* 33, no. 4
(October 13, 2023): 326–29, https://doi.org/10.5152/pcp.2023.23690; and
Alan D. Kaye et al., "Efficacy and Safety of Alpha-2 Agonists in Autism
Spectrum Disorder: A Systematic Review," *Advances in Therapy* 41, no. 11
(September 13, 2024): 4299–311, https://doi.org/10.1007/s12325-024
-02980-0.

31. Althea A. Robinson and Beth A. Malow, "Gabapentin Shows Promise in
Treating Refractory Insomnia in Children," *Journal of Child Neurology* 28,
no. 12 (October 30, 2012): 1618–21, https://doi.org/10.1177/088307381
2463069.

32. Salam Salloum-Asfar, Nasser Zawia, and Sara A. Abdulla, "Retracing
Our Steps: A Review on Autism Research in Children, Its Limitation and
Impending Pharmacological Interventions," *Pharmacology & Therapeutics*
253 (January 2024): 108564, https://doi.org/10.1016/j.pharmthera
.2023.108564.

Chapter 19: Nothing Is Working! What Else Is There?

1. A. J. P. Francis and R. J. W. Dempster, "Effect of Valerian, *Valeriana Edulis*,
on Sleep Difficulties in Children with Intellectual Deficits: Randomised
Trial," *Phytomedicine* 9, no. 4 (January 2002): 273–79, https://doi.org
/10.1078/0944-7113-00110.

2. William G. Sharp et al., "Dietary Intake, Nutrient Status, and Growth
Parameters in Children with Autism Spectrum Disorder and Severe Food
Selectivity: An Electronic Medical Record Review," *Journal of the Academy
of Nutrition and Dietetics* 118, no. 10 (October 2018): 1943–50, https://doi
.org/10.1016/j.jand.2018.05.005.

3. Patricia A. Stewart et al., "Dietary Supplementation in Children with
Autism Spectrum Disorders: Common, Insufficient, and Excessive,"
Journal of the Academy of Nutrition and Dietetics 115, no. 8 (August 2015):
1237–48, https://doi.org/10.1016/j.jand.2015.03.026.

4. Swapna N. Deshpande and Deborah R. Simkin, "Complementary and Integrative Approaches to Sleep Disorders in Children," *Child and Adolescent
Psychiatric Clinics of North America* 32, no. 2 (April 2023): 243–72, https://
doi.org/10.1016/j.chc.2022.08.008.

5. Meritxell Rojo-Marticella, Victoria Arija, and Josefa Canals-Sans, "Effect
of Probiotics on the Symptomatology of Autism Spectrum Disorder and/
or Attention Deficit/Hyperactivity Disorder in Children and Adolescents:
Pilot Study," *Research on Child and Adolescent Psychopathology* 53, no. 2
(January 11, 2025): 163–78, https://doi.org/10.1007/s10802-024-01278-7.

6. Elena Zambrelli et al., "Effects of Supplementation with Antioxidant

Agents on Sleep in Autism Spectrum Disorder: A Review," *Frontiers in Psychiatry* 12 (June 28, 2021), https://doi.org/10.3389/fpsyt.2021.689277; and Elham Mousavinejad et al., "Coenzyme Q10 Supplementation Reduces Oxidative Stress and Decreases Antioxidant Enzyme Activity in Children with Autism Spectrum Disorders," *Psychiatry Research* 265 (July 2018): 62–69, https://doi.org/10.1016/j.psychres.2018.03.061.

7. F. N. U. Abhishek et al., "Dietary Interventions and Supplements for Managing Attention-Deficit/Hyperactivity Disorder (ADHD): A Systematic Review of Efficacy and Recommendations," *Cureus*, September 20, 2024, https://doi.org/10.7759/cureus.69804; and Susan L. Hyman at al., "The Gluten-Free/Casein-Free Diet: A Double-Blind Challenge Trial in Children with Autism," *Journal of Autism and Developmental Disorders* 46, no. 1 (September 5, 2015): 205–20, https://doi.org/10.1007/s10803-015-2564-9.

8. Julie S. Matthews and James B. Adams, "Ratings of the Effectiveness of 13 Therapeutic Diets for Autism Spectrum Disorder: Results of a National Survey," *Journal of Personalized Medicine* 13, no. 10 (September 29, 2023): 1448, https://doi.org/10.3390/jpm13101448.

9. Dawson et al., "Weighted Blankets as a Sleep Intervention" (chap. 16, n. 7).

10. Lisa Mische Lawson et al., "Exploring Effects of Sensory Garments on Participation of Children on the Autism Spectrum: A Pretest-Posttest Repeated Measure Design," *Occupational Therapy International* (June 6, 2022): 3540271, https://doi.org/10.1155/2022/3540271.

11. Xiaobin Ge et al., "Tiny Needles, Major Benefits: Acupuncture in Child Health," *BMC Pediatrics* 25, no. 1 (April 14, 2025), https://doi.org/10.1186/s12887-025-05586-9.

12. Daniel K. L. Cheuk et al., "Acupuncture for Insomnia," *Cochrane Database of Systematic Reviews* 2012, no. 9 (September 12, 2012), https://doi.org/10.1002/14651858.cd005472.pub3.

13. Annabelle Snow, Jaime Ralston-Wilson, and Ryan Milley, "Acupuncture in Pediatrics: A Scoping Review," *Journal of Integrative and Complementary Medicine* 31, no. 4 (April 1, 2025): 335–49, https://doi.org/10.1089/jicm.2024.0150; and Peter Gilbey et al., "Acupuncture for Posttonsillectomy Pain in Children: A Randomized, Controlled Study," *Pediatric Anesthesia* 25, no. 6 (February 7, 2015): 603–9, https://doi.org/10.1111/pan.12621.

14. Fei-Yi Zhao et al., "Is Integrating Acupuncture into the Management of Attention-Deficit/Hyperactivity Disorder Among Children and Adolescents Now Opportune and Evidence-Based? A Systematic Review with Meta-Analysis and Trial Sequential Analysis," *Complementary Therapies in Medicine* 90 (June 2025): 103163, https://doi.org/10.1016/j.ctim.2025.103163.

15. Aníbal Báez-Suárez et al., "Application of Non-Invasive Neuromodulation in Children with Neurodevelopmental Disorders to Improve Their Sleep Quality and Constipation," *BMC Pediatrics* 23, no. 1 (September 15, 2023), https://doi.org/10.1186/s12887-023-04307-4.

16. Juan Yan et al., "Effects of Transcranial Magnetic Stimulation on Sleep

Structure and Quality in Children with Autism," *Frontiers in Psychiatry* 15 (June 28, 2024), https://doi.org/10.3389/fpsyt.2024.1413961.

17. Lei Gao et al., "The Sensory Abnormality Mediated Partially the Efficacy of Repetitive Transcranial Magnetic Stimulation on Treating Comorbid Sleep Disorder in Autism Spectrum Disorder Children," *Frontiers in Psychiatry* 12 (January 24, 2022), https://doi.org/10.3389/fpsyt.2021.820598.

18. Nianyi Sun et al., "The Effect of Repetitive Transcranial Magnetic Stimulation for Insomnia: A Systematic Review and Meta-Analysis," *Sleep Medicine* 77 (January 2021): 226–37, https://doi.org/10.1016/j.sleep.2020.05.020.

19. Igor Val Danilov, "The Origin of Natural Neurostimulation: A Narrative Review of Noninvasive Brain Stimulation Techniques," *OBM Neurobiology* 8, no. 4 (November 29, 2024): 1–23, https://doi.org/10.21926/obm.neurobiol.2404260.

20. Shanthi Krishnaswami, Melissa L. McPheeters, and Jeremy Veenstra-VanderWeele. "A Systematic Review of Secretin for Children with Autism Spectrum Disorders," *Pediatrics* 127, no. 5 (May 1, 2011), https://doi.org/10.1542/peds.2011-0428.

Chapter 20: Teen Sleep Is a Different Animal

1. Rebecca Robbins et al., "Adolescent Sleep Myths: Identifying False Beliefs That Impact Adolescent Sleep and Well-Being," *Sleep Health* 8, no. 9 (September 2012), https://doi.org/10.1016/j.sleh.2022.08.001.

2. Kate A. Bartel, Michael Gradisar, and Paul Williamson, "Protective and Risk Factors for Adolescent Sleep: A Meta-Analytic Review," *Sleep Medicine Reviews* 21 (June 2015): 72–85, https://doi.org/10.1016/j.smrv.2014.08.002.

3. Beth Malow et al., "Trajectory of Sleep Patterns Across Adolescence in Autistic and Neurotypical Youth," *SLEEP* 48, no. Supplement 1 (May 2025), https://doi.org/10.1093/sleep/zsaf090.1053.

4. Pavlopoulou, "Good Night's Sleep" (chap. 16, n. 8).

Chapter 21: What About the Rest of the Family?

1. Kailey E. Penner et al., "'Bottom of My Own List': Barriers and Facilitators to Mental Health Support Use in Caregivers of Children with Neurodevelopmental Support Needs," *Journal of Autism and Developmental Disorders* (June 2024), https://doi.org/10.1007/s10803-024-06409-z.

2. Candice Luo, "A Comparison of Electronically-Delivered and Face to Face Cognitive Behavioural Therapies in Depressive Disorders: A Systematic Review and Meta-Analysis," *EClinicalMedicine* 24 (July 2020): 100442, https://doi.org/10.1016/j.eclinm.2020.100442.

3. Cynthia R. Johnson et al., "Telehealth Parent Training for Sleep

Disturbances in Young Children with Autism Spectrum Disorder: A Randomized Controlled Trial," *Sleep Medicine* 111 (November 2023): 208–19, https://doi.org/10.1016/j.sleep.2023.08.033.

4. Brooke K. Iwamoto et al., "Exploring Bidirectional Relationships: Child Sleep Duration, Child Behavior Problems, and Parenting Stress in Families of Children with Autism Spectrum Disorder," *Research in Autism Spectrum Disorders* 106 (August 2023): 102197, https://doi.org/10.1016/j.rasd.2023.102197.

5. L. J. Meltzer, "Brief Report: Sleep in Parents of Children with Autism Spectrum Disorders," *Journal of Pediatric Psychology* 33, no. 4 (May 2008): 380–86, https://doi.org/10.1093/jpepsy/jsn005.

6. S. Gallagher, A. C. Phillips, and D. Carroll, "Parental Stress Is Associated with Poor Sleep Quality in Parents Caring for Children with Developmental Disabilities," *Journal of Pediatric Psychology* 35, no. 7 (October 29, 2009): 728–37, https://doi.org/10.1093/jpepsy/jsp093.

7. S. Gallagher et al., "Predictors of Psychological Morbidity in Parents of Children with Intellectual Disabilities," *Journal of Pediatric Psychology* 33, no. 10 (February 4, 2008): 1129–36, https://doi.org/10.1093/jpepsy/jsn040.

8. Kenneth Curley, Robert Hughes, and Yasuhiro Kotera, "Stressful but Not Unhappy: A Review of the Positive Aspects of Parenting a Child with Autism Spectrum Disorder," *Children* 12, no. 1 (January 17, 2025): 107, https://doi.org/10.3390/children12010107.

9. Georgia Pavlopoulou et al., "'Who Listens to the Listener, Who Cares for the Carer?': A Cross-Sectional Study of Social Connectedness and Sleep Experiences of Young Siblings of Neurodivergent People," *Child: Care, Health and Development* 51 (December 3, 2024), https://doi.org/10.31234/osf.io/kvy5d.

10. Georgia Pavlopoulou et al., "'I Often Have to Explain to School Staff What She Needs': School Experiences of Non-Autistic Siblings Growing Up with an Autistic Brother or Sister," *Research in Developmental Disabilities* 129 (October 2022): 104323, https://doi.org/10.1016/j.ridd.2022.104323.

11. Emma Cooke et al., "Siblings' Experiences of Sleep Disruption in Families with a Child with Down Syndrome," *Sleep Health* 10, no. 2 (April 2024): 198–204, https://doi.org/10.1016/j.sleh.2023.10.002.

Resources

American Academy of Sleep Medicine: www.sleepeducation.org
Autism Speaks Sleep Toolkit: www.autismspeaks.org/sleep
Hope Grows for Autism: www.hopegrowsforautism.org
National Sleep Foundation: www.thensf.org
Pediatric Sleep Council: www.babysleep.com
Project Sleep: www.project-sleep.com
Society for Behavioral Sleep Medicine: www.behavioralsleep.org

Index

Page references followed by an italicized *t.* indicate tables.

About the Author

Melisa Moore, PhD, loves sleep and helping others get more of it. A clinical psychologist board certified in behavioral sleep medicine, she works for the Sleep Center at Rady Children's Health. She also maintains a private practice supporting children, teens, and young adults across the country with a variety of sleep and mood issues. Previously, Dr. Moore served on the faculty at the University of Pennsylvania and was the Psychosocial Director of the Sleep Center at Children's Hospital of Philadelphia (CHOP). She now lives with her husband and two sons in the Los Angeles area, where she continues to believe in the power of a good night's sleep. For more, visit www.drmelisamoore.com.